Investigating and Managing Common Cardiovascular Conditions

Juan Carlos Kaski
Michael Papadakis
Hariharan Raju
Editors

Investigating and Managing Common Cardiovascular Conditions

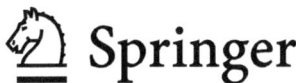 Springer

Editors
Juan Carlos Kaski
Cardiac Research Centre
St George's University
of London
London
UK

Hariharan Raju
Cardiac Research Centre
St George's University
of London
London
UK

Michael Papadakis
Cardiac Research Centre
St George's University
of London
London
UK

ISBN 978-1-4471-6695-5   ISBN 978-1-4471-6696-2   (eBook)
DOI 10.1007/978-1-4471-6696-2

Library of Congress Control Number: 2015949239

Springer London Heidelberg New York Dordrecht

Printed on acid-free paper

Springer-Verlag London Ltd. is part of Springer Science+Business Media
(www.springer.com)

Foreword

Junior doctors find the likelihood of being allocated to a post involving cardiology a gratifying and thrilling but somewhat frightening prospect. It is well known that cardiology is a discipline which deals with acute life-and-death situations, where errors cannot be tolerated. Many young doctors face cardiology posts with "shivers up the spine". Fortunately this concern has now been recognised by the editors and authors of this new handbook. Five potentially terrifying presentations have been identified and their management has been laid out in a simple and straightforward fashion. The format is novel: the section is written primarily by a trainee – closely aligned to the practical problem – and overviewed by a senior cardiologist with substantial experience in each of the presentations. This provides a valuable blend of practice and theory which is crucial to the doctor who is "on the spot". The text is concise and easy to read – it is enormously valuable to those who have to cope with immediate problems. It is both practical and sound from a theoretical perspective – it is good value for the time invested in giving it your attention.

London, UK   A. John Camm

Preface

This clinical handbook aims to serve as a practical guide for general practitioners, cardiology trainees, nurses with an interest in cardiology, and junior physicians, in general, who face the challenge of assisting people affected by cardiovascular conditions. We envisage our colleagues using this book as a quick reference in everyday clinical practice but also when they wish to remind themselves of key diagnostic elements and current management strategies for common – but often problematic – cardiovascular conditions. As such, we have, in the present handbook, focused on those cardiovascular conditions that clinicians are likely to encounter more frequently in their practice and which pose major diagnostic and therapeutic challenges.

The chapters in the book, which have all been written by cardiology trainees under the direct supervision of a senior author with particular expertise in the field, have been structured in a fashion that we believe will provide the reader with a truly practical tool. We have hopefully addressed most of the questions commonly asked in relation to the diagnosis, differential diagnoses and management of the cardiovascular conditions presented in the book. Given the practical nature of the handbook we have incorporated sections such as "Must do's" and "Red flags" to help the reader in dealing rapidly and efficiently with the most relevant clinical issues.

We have placed emphasis on the pharmacological treatment of the conditions mentioned in the handbook, and to the best of our knowledge all the information contained in the chapters is evidence-based. Flowcharts, diagrams and images have been included to facilitate the reading of the book.

We truly hope that you will enjoy reading the handbook and find it to be a useful tool to assist you in your clinical endeavours and will be delighted if our work contributes to benefit patients accordingly.

London, UK   Juan Carlos Kaski
                                           Michael Papadakis
                                            Hariharan Raju

Acknowledgements

We would like to express our gratitude to all contributing authors for their hard work and dedication in making this book a reality.

Contents

Contributors

Editors

Juan Carlos Kaski Cardiovascular Sciences Research Centre, Cardiovascular and Cell Sciences Research Institute, St George's University of London, London, UK

Michael Papadakis Cardiovascular Sciences Research Centre, Cardiovascular and Cell Sciences Research Institute, St George's University of London, London, UK

Hariharan Raju Cardiovascular Sciences Research Centre, Cardiovascular and Cell Sciences Research Institute, St George's University of London, London, UK

Contributors

Elijah R. Behr, MA, MBBS, MD, FRCP Cardiovascular Sciences Research Centre, Cardiovascular and Cell Sciences Research Institute, St George's University of London, London, UK

Teck K. Khong, FRCP, MD, MBA Blood Pressure Unit, St George's Hospital NHS Trust, London, UK

Institute of Medical & Biomedical Education, St George's University of London, London, UK

Anthony Li, MBBS, MRCP Cardiovascular Sciences Research Centre, Cardiovascular and Cell Sciences Research Institute, St George's University of London, London, UK

Jayesh Makan, BSc (Hons), MBBS Department of Cardiology, Shrewsbury and Telford NHS Trust, Shrewsbury, UK

Lynne Millar, MB BCh, BAO, MRCP Cardiovascular Sciences Research Centre, Cardiovascular and Cell Sciences Research Institute, St George's University of London, London, UK

Jennifer Roe, MBBS Blood Pressure Unit, St George's Hospital NHS Trust, London, UK

Magdi M. Saba, MD, FHRS Cardiac Electrophysiology, St. George's Hospital and University of London, London, UK

Sanjay Sharma, BSc(Hons), MBChB, MD, FRCP, FESC Cardiovascular Sciences Research Centre, Cardiovascular and Cell Sciences Research Institute, St George's University of London, London, UK

Kostas Zacharias Department of Cardiology, Barts Heart Centre, London, UK

Chapter 1
Chest Pain

Kostas Zacharias and Jayesh Makan

Introduction

Patients presenting with chest pain account for over 500,000 primary care appointments per year and for up to 25 % of attendances in Emergency Departments in the UK. The spectrum of diagnoses in patients presenting with chest pain ranges from acute life threatening conditions such as acute myocardial infarction, aortic dissection and pulmonary embolism to benign conditions such as musculoskeletal disorders. The timely and accurate diagnosis of such patients therefore remains a challenge for all physicians. The aim of this chapter is to provide guidance regarding the differential diagnosis in a patient presenting with chest pain with emphasis on the diagnosis and management of myocardial ischaemia.

K. Zacharias
Department of Cardiology, Barts Heart Centre,
London EC1A 7BE, UK
e-mail: kzacharias23@hotmail.com

J. Makan, BSc (Hons), MBBS (✉)
Department of Cardiology, Shrewsbury and Telford NHS Trust,
Shrewsbury SY3 8XQ, UK
e-mail: jayeshmakan@btinternet.com

J.C. Kaski et al. (eds.), *Investigating and Managing Common Cardiovascular Conditions*, DOI 10.1007/978-1-4471-6696-2_1,
© Springer-Verlag London 2015

Differential Diagnosis

Chest pain can be the presenting symptom in a range of conditions. The most important causes of chest pain are shown in Table 1.1. Acute Coronary Syndrome (ACS) is the final diagnosis in only 15–25 % of patients who present with acute chest pain. Nevertheless, the diagnosis of ACS in such patients may still be missed, with potentially life-threatening results. A detailed history and systematic use of basic investigations can aid the non-specialist in correctly identifying patients with ACS and referring them appropriately for specialist management.

Initial Assessment of the Patient

In the acute setting, initial assessment may take place prior to physician contact, with paramedics or nurses triaging individuals. A 12-lead electrocardiogram (ECG) should be recorded and assessed at the earliest possible opportunity, preferably within 10 min, in all patients who present with ongoing chest pain of suspected cardiac origin. The priority is to address whether the patient is clinically stable or at risk of a life-threatening condition such as ACS, aortic dissection or pulmonary embolism. If not critically ill, a decision regarding urgency for further investigation must be made by risk-stratifying patients. Patients who display ST segment elevation on their ECG must be triaged as critical priorities and directed to specialist cardiology centres with a view to cardiac catheterisation as an emergency.

   The diagnosis and assessment of a patient with suspected stable angina involves a comprehensive clinical evaluation, including identifying significant dyslipidaemia, hyperglycaemia or other biochemical risk factors and specific cardiac investigations. These investigations may be used to confirm the diagnosis of ischaemia, to identify or exclude associated conditions or precipitating factors, assist in risk stratifying patients and to evaluate the efficacy of treatment (Fig. 1.1).

TABLE 1.1 Most common causes of chest pain

Category	Syndrome	Key features
Cardiac	Stable angina	Precipitated by exertion/ relieved by rest
	Acute coronary syndromes	Sudden onset/duration >20 min. Associated with dyspnoea and autonomic symptoms
	Pericarditis	Sharp, pleuritic. Relieved by leaning forwards
Respiratory	Pneumothorax	Unilateral. Pleuritic. Sudden onset
	Pleuritis/ pneumonia	Pleuritic/infective symptoms
Vascular	Aortic dissection	Very severe/radiating to the back
	Pulmonary embolism	Pleuritic/dyspnoea
Gastrointestinal	Gastro- oesophageal reflux	Following large meal/ relieved by antacid
	Peptic ulcer disease	Relieved by antacid
	Pancreatitis	Intense epigastric/ substernal
	Gallbladder disease	Usually following fatty meal
Musculoskeletal	Costochondritis	Reproduced on palpation
	Trauma	History of trauma
Neurological	Cervical spine pathology	Reproduced by neck movement
Infectious	Herpes zoster	Burning/dermatomal distribution
Psychological	Panic attack	Hyperventilation

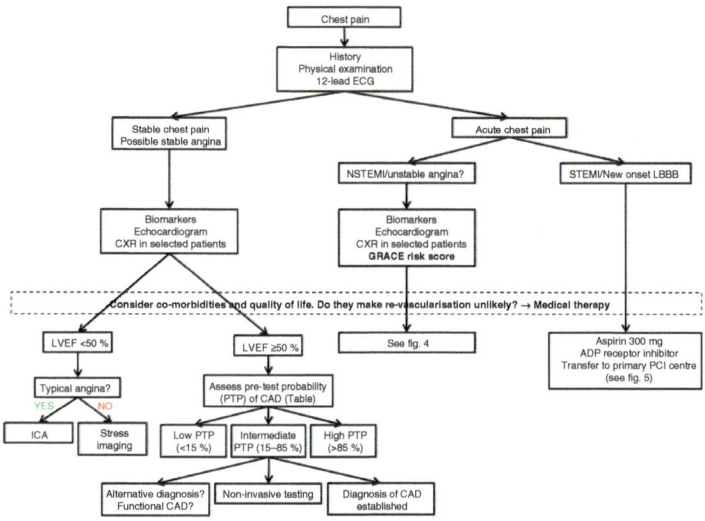

FIGURE 1.1 Initial diagnostic management of patients presenting with chest pain. *ADP* adenosine diphosphate, *ICA* invasive coronary angiography, *LVEF* left ventricular ejection fraction

History

The classic manifestation of pain that is caused by myocardial ischaemia is angina. This may be described amongst other things as dull discomfort, crushing sensation, restriction, "band-like" sensation or throat tightness. The discomfort is classically brought on by physical or in some cases emotional stress and may radiate into the jaw, one or both shoulders or arms (though not to fingertips).

A description of central chest pain that is brought on by exercise and relieved by rest or by the use of glyceryl trinitrate (GTN) is thought to constitute typical angina. By contrast the following descriptions of pain make the diagnosis of angina less likely:

(a) pain that is primarily pleuritic
(b) pain that is entirely in the abdomen

(c) pain that can be localized by the patient with the use of one finger

(d) pain that lasts for a few seconds or pain that persists for many hours or days

(e) pain that can be reproduced by movement or palpation of the chest or of the arms

In general, patients with symptoms of chest discomfort, dyspnoea or dizziness that are clearly related to exertion should be referred for further assessment with regards to underlying coronary artery disease (CAD).

Risk Factors

The main risk factors for ischaemic heart disease are well described in various population studies. Non-modifiable risk factors include increasing age and male gender; male patients over the age of 70 have over 90 % probability of underlying CAD even when presenting with atypical pain (Table 1.2).

Amongst the modifiable risk factors, diabetes mellitus, smoking status and hyperlipidaemia confer a higher predictive value than hypertension. Familial premature CAD (below age 55 years in a male non-smoker, below 65 years in a female), usually occurs in the context of other risk factors such as familial dyslipidaemia and thus, on its own, does not confer as high a predictive value as previously thought.

It should be noted that this risk factor profiling applies to patients with no previous diagnosis of CAD, i.e. only at the time of index presentation. Any patient with a prior myocardial infarction (MI), demonstrable CAD on coronary angiography or prior coronary revascularization has an established diagnosis of CAD. Thus, chest discomfort in such patients should be thoroughly evaluated. Risk factor modification in such patients is important for their prognosis and prevention of recurrent cardiovascular events.

TABLE 1.2 Clinical pre-test probability in patients with stable chest pain symptoms

Age (yrs)	Typical angina		Atypical angina		Non-anginal pain	
	Male	Female	Male	Female	Male	Female
30–39	59	28	29	10	18	5
40–49	69	37	38	14	25	8
50–59	77	47	49	20	34	12
60–69	84	58	59	28	44	17
70–79	89	68	69	37	54	24
>80	93	76	78	47	65	32

Adapted from 2013 ESC guidelines on the management of stable coronary artery disease. Eur Heart J. 2013;34:2949–3003

Values are % of people at each mid-decade age with significant coronary artery disease (CAD)

Probability < 15 % can be managed without further testing

Probability of 15–65 % should have a non-invasive imaging based test for ischaemia, allowing for local expertise and availability. In young patients radiation issues should be considered. An exercise ECG is an alternative as the initial test

Probability between 66 and 85 % should have a non-invasive imaging functional test for making a diagnosis of CAD

Probability of >85 % one can assume that CAD is present. They need risk stratification only

Physical Examination

A thorough examination of the cardiovascular and respiratory system should be performed in all patients. Although there are no pathognomonic physical signs of CAD, a physical examination may reveal signs that point towards alternative diagnoses. These may include signs of:

(i) systemic conditions/illnesses (e.g. sepsis, anaemia, thyroid disease, generalized malignancy)
(ii) other heart disease (e.g. murmur of aortic stenosis or hypertrophic cardiomyopathy, friction rub of pericarditis)

(iii) vascular disease (e.g. difference in arm blood pressures indicating aortic dissection, signs of pulmonary hypertension in pulmonary embolism)

(iv) respiratory disease (e.g. signs of pneumonia, pleural rub, signs of pneumothorax)

Investigations

ECG

A 12-lead ECG should be obtained and interpreted at presentation. The following criteria constitute acute transmural ischaemia, consistent with the diagnosis of ST elevation myocardial infarction (STEMI) in a patient presenting with symptoms of chest pain and should prompt urgent specialist referral:

ST elevation of ≥2 mm in at least two contiguous precordial leads (V1-V6)

ST elevation of ≥1 mm in at least two limb leads of same territory (lateral: I, aVL; inferior: II, III, aVF)

Left bundle branch block (LBBB) that is not known to be old

ST-depression in leads V1-V3 with associated dominant R-wave (suggestive of isolated posterior STEMI) (Fig. 1.2)

ST-segment elevation in lead aVR, particularly when associated with precordial lead ST depression is suggestive of left main stem ischaemia (Fig. 1.3)

The presence of a ventricular paced rhythm and LBBB make interpretation of the ECG for evidence of acute ischaemia challenging. In such cases, patients with ongoing symptoms suggestive of myocardial ischaemia, such as persistent chest pain, autonomic symptoms (sweating and nausea), signs of acute heart failure or impending shock also deserve prompt specialist assessment. It's also important to remember that a normal ECG does not rule out an acute coronary event!

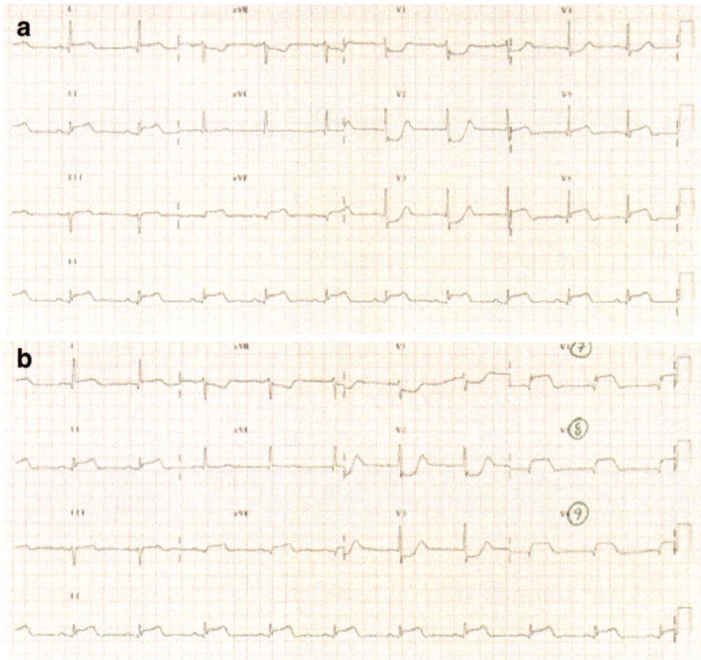

FIGURE 1.2 (**a**) ECG demonstrating an infero-postero-lateral STEMI in a patient with acute chest pain. Note the presence of ST-depression in leads V1-V3 with associated dominant R-wave. (**b**) Placing leads V4-V6 posteriorly (V7-V9) unmasks the posterior ST-elevation

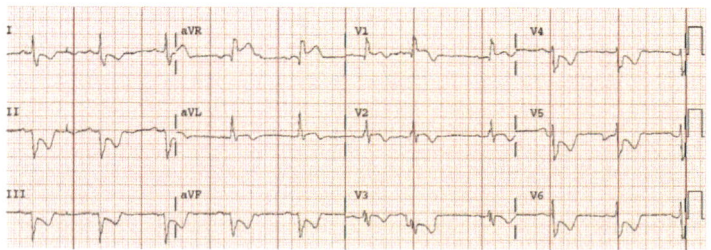

FIGURE 1.3 ECG demonstrating ST-segment elevation in lead aVR, with associated ST depression in the precordial leads, suggestive of left main stem ischaemia

Patients with ECG abnormalities that do not fall into any of the categories detailed above are not thought to benefit from early reperfusion therapy. However patients with clearly dynamic ECG changes (dynamic ST depression that occurs during episodes of chest pain or progressive T-wave inversion and deepening) may be considered for early coronary angiography.

ECG rhythm monitoring should be initiated as soon as possible in all patients with suspected STEMI and continue for at least 24 h after successful reperfusion therapy due to the risk of acute ischaemic or early post-MI ventricular arrhythmia.

Myocardial Biomarkers

The use of biomarkers in the diagnosis of myocardial ischaemia has changed considerably over recent years. The diagnosis of myocardial infarction was initially reliant on assays of creatine kinase (CK), its iso-enzyme (CK-MB) and myoglobin. Although useful, they were limited by low sensitivity and specificity. The advent of troponin assays allowed for greater diagnostic accuracy and thus troponin is now the biomarker of choice for detecting myocardial damage. In patients with a myocardial infarction, levels may be elevated as early as 4 h after the event and can remain elevated for up to 2 weeks. A troponin assay may therefore also be of value in the assessment of patients who present late. High sensitivity troponin assays provide even greater sensitivity and by using serial samples, for example 3 h apart, the sensitivity for diagnosing MI approaches 100 %. Current guidance advocates a troponin sampling at admission and repeat measurement between 10 and 12 h after the onset of symptoms. This provides the opportunity to assess the pattern of change. The progression from the first to second sample is important as it may help to differentiate acute infarction from chronic myocardial necrosis.

It is important to note that troponin should not be used as the sole investigation to diagnose or exclude ACS. The history,

TABLE 1.3 Causes of raised troponin levels (apart from ACS)

1. Pulmonary embolism

2. Congestive heart failure

3. Arrhythmias

4. Septicaemia

5. Myocarditis

6. Neurological conditions e.g. subarachnoid haemorrhage

7. Aortic dissection

8. Iatrogenic e.g. pacing, electrophysiological studies

9. Chronic or acute kidney injury

10. Infiltrative disease e.g. sarcoidosis, haemochromatosis

11. Drugs e.g. chemotherapy

clinical findings and ECG remain the cornerstone of the diagnostic process. Troponin levels may be elevated in response to other pathologies (Table 1.3) and one must be prepared to consider an alternative diagnosis as suggested by the history and clinical examination findings.

Other biomarker assays have been evaluated. These include myeloperoxidase and ischaemia modified albumin. Their value in clinical practice over high-sensitivity troponin has not yet been established. Measurement of B-type Natriuretic Peptide (BNP) levels provides useful prognostic information but should not be used to determine initial therapeutic strategies in ACS. Similarly, high sensitivity CRP can predict long-term mortality but is of limited use in acute cardiac presentations.

Functional Imaging

There are various testing modalities that try to look for objective evidence of functional ischaemia in patients who present with stable symptoms.

The exercise ECG (ExECG), also referred to as an exercise tolerance test, has been used for a number of years as the investigation of choice in most of these patients. Although, it retains its Class I recommendation in guidelines from the USA, it is no longer recommended as the first-line screening test for functional ischaemia in the UK and the rest of Europe. Its main advantage of widespread availability has been overshadowed by the high number of inconclusive tests, approximately 30 % in most studies. Its role is now limited to the assessment of exercise capacity in patients with established CAD. Allowing for availability of local expertise and resources, alternative stress imaging modalities such as echocardiogram, cardiac magnetic resonance imaging (CMR), single photon emission computed tomography (SPECT) or positron emission tomography (PET) are recommended in patients with suspected but stable CAD with intermediate pre-test probability, as first line investigation. Clinician and patient preference also dictate the choice of test.

Stress echocardiography is a well-established functional assessment modality. It provides real-time information on cardiac structure and function, coupled with a high degree of sensitivity and specificity for CAD. Patients who are unable to exercise can undergo assessment with a pharmacological stressor such as dobutamine. The introduction of echocardiographic contrast media has improved endocardial definition to the point where a diagnostic-standard test can be performed in all but a very small minority of patients.

Nuclear myocardial perfusion study (MPS), including SPECT and PET, is another well-established functional imaging technique. It has a comparable sensitivity and specificity to stress echocardiography. Its main disadvantages include the need for specialized equipment and the involvement of ionizing radiation. It can also underestimate the severity of CAD in the context of balanced ischaemia, such as seen in three-vessel disease.

Cardiac magnetic resonance (CMR) imaging is developing into a viable alternative assessment for functional ischaemia. However, this imaging modality is not yet widely available and its cost may limit its widespread use in the future. Its main benefit is the additional anatomical information provided, which is accepted as surpassing that of echocardiography.

Anatomical Imaging

Invasive coronary angiography is considered the gold-standard for investigation of epicardial coronary artery disease. At present, it is considered as a first-line investigation for stable angina in individuals with a high pre-test probability of CAD (>85 %) where revascularisation is being considered. It is also appropriate for further evaluation of functional ischaemia on non-invasive investigations as a prelude to revascularisation, which may take place at the same time. The risks of invasive coronary angiography should be taken into account, which include vascular damage and systemic thromboembolic phenomena.

Computed tomography coronary angiography (CTCA) is now available as a non-invasive anatomical test. Its main use at present is in patients with low or low-intermediate pre-test probability (10–50 %) of CAD as a rule-out test. The advance of technology has significantly limited the amount of radiation involved. A CTCA can also be performed to delineate the course of anomalous coronary vessels or grafted vessels in patients with a previous history of coronary bypass surgery.

Management

NSTEMI and Unstable Angina

Patients who present with cardiac chest pain occurring at rest, or minimal exertion and that is not responsive to a short acting nitrate should be treated as unstable. Patients with angina of recent onset that occurs at decreasing levels of exertion (crescendo angina) should also be considered unstable.

TABLE 1.4 Risk assessment of ACS patients (GRACE Score, adapted from NICE Clinical guideline 94)

Predicted 6 month mortality	Risk of future adverse cardiovascular events
<1.5 %	Very low risk
>1.5–3 %	Low risk
>3–6 %	Intermediate risk
>6–9 %	High risk
>9 %	Highest risk

As with any critically ill patient, respiratory and haemodynamic assessment should triage direction and urgency of further assessment. The patient should have cardiac monitoring instituted with intravenous access obtained. Often, local institutions have departmental policies for management of ACS. However, the priority is to establish a hierarchy of differential diagnoses prior to initiation of any treatment, since treatments targeted at ACS, such as aggressive antiplatelet agents, may be deleterious in other conditions.

The overall mortality and morbidity risk of patients with suspected ACS should be calculated early on and taken into consideration when further therapy is decided. Current clinical guidelines recommend quantitative assessment with the use of a scoring system such as the GRACE or TIMI scores. An online calculator for the GRACE score is accessible at www.outcomes-umassmed.org/grace/acs_risk/acs_risk_content.html. The GRACE score provides an estimation for the probability of death or myocardial infarction both in-hospital and at 6 months. This calculation can help the clinician to tailor treatment accordingly. Patients can be categorized on the basis of their GRACE score (Table 1.4) to low, intermediate or high risk. It is worth noting that a patient with dynamic ECG changes and a negative troponin has an equal or greater risk than a patient of similar characteristics with no ECG changes and a positive troponin. This further illustrates the pitfall of basing ACS diagnosis and management on the troponin value alone.

The overall risk/benefit ratio with regards to potential bleeding complications in an individual patient should also be assessed. Online tools such as the Crusade bleeding score (www.crusadebleedingscore.org) are easily accessible and can be used to calculate the risk of in-hospital major bleeding.

Symptomatic Treatments

Appropriate analgesia will render the patient more comfortable and should therefore be initiated early. Systemic nitrates, such as glyceryl trinitrate (GTN), are rapidly absorbed sublingually or bucally. Alternatively, they also come in intravenous preparations for continuous infusion for ongoing pain. They act by coronary vasodilation, thereby improving subendocardial ischaemia. Opioids such as morphine or diamorphine may be required and administration is usually combined with that of an antiemetic such as metoclopramide. Resultant vasodilation from these treatments may rarely precipitate hypotension, though cardiogenic shock must be considered in this context. Universal use of high flow oxygen is not warranted unless the oxygen saturations are low (less than 94 %).

Antiplatelet/Antithrombin Therapy

A wide variety of drugs are available in this category of therapeutic agent and local guidance, if available, should be consulted. We have presented here an overview of available options and factors that may favour one agent over another.

A loading dose of 150–300 mg aspirin (acetylsalicylic acid) should be given in suspected ACS, unless there is a clear history of significant aspirin allergy. It is important to note that patients may state that they are allergic to aspirin on the basis of a mild gastric upset or asthma. In such cases, aspirin should still be offered. In definite systemic, respiratory or cutaneous sensitivity reactions to prior aspirin use, however, monotherapy with another antiplatelet agent such as an adenosine diphosphate (ADP) receptor inhibitor should be considered.

An ADP receptor inhibitor such as clopidogrel (300–600 mg loading dose, 75 mg daily maintenance dose), ticagrelor (180 mg loading dose, 90 mg twice-daily maintenance dose) or prasugrel (60 mg loading dose, 10 mg daily maintenance dose) should be co-administered with aspirin. The latter two newer agents, are now recommended as first choice as they carry a better ischaemic prognosis, albeit at somewhat higher risk of bleeding events. Additionally, the newer agents have more predictable antiplatelet effects. Based on the ESC guidelines, ticagrelor, is recommended for all patients at moderate to high risk of ischaemic events including those pre-treated with clopidogrel, which should be discontinued when ticagrelor is commenced. Prasugrel on the other hand should be considered in ADP-inhibitor naïve patients, particularly diabetics, in whom the coronary anatomy is known and who are proceeding to coronary intervention (PCI).

Anticoagulation is recommended for all patients in addition to anti-platelet therapy. It should be selected according to both ischaemic and bleeding risks and according to the efficacy and safety profile of individual agents. Unfractionated heparin, low molecular weight heparins (such as enoxaparin or dalteparin), and fondaparinux (a more selective anti-factor Xa agent) reduce recurrent ischaemic events and overall mortality. Fondaparinux 2.5 mg subcutaneously is recommended as first choice as it has the most favourable efficacy-safety profile with the most favourable bleeding profile. Unfractionated heparin may be preferred in those with end-stage kidney disease; dose reduction and/or adjustment may be necessary if low molecular weight drugs or fondaparinux are used in those with renal impairment or when used over prolonged periods.

In very high-risk patients, the addition of other anti-platelet agents such as glycoprotein IIb/IIIa inhibitor (GPI –eg Tirofiban, Eptifibatide) should be considered, with combination of GPI. The combination of GPI and heparin analogue or GPI with bivalirudin if the benefit of giving these agents is thought to outweigh the potential extra bleeding risk. The latter has a better bleeding profile and is considered appropriate for those at high ischaemic and high bleeding risk.

Patients at low risk can be managed conservatively in the first instance but should still be offered a non-invasive functional test for ischaemia prior to discharge from hospital. It is important to remember that when considering absolute numbers, the majority of subsequent coronary events occur in patients deemed at low risk. This is because, numerically, these patients represent the overwhelmingly largest group of presentations. It is therefore important to accurately further risk stratify these patients by means of a functional test prior to discharge. Invasive investigation with angiography should be reserved for those with demonstrable inducible ischaemia on functional testing.

Urgent discussion and referral to a specialist should take place in the cases of patients who suffer from haemodynamic instability, acute left ventricular dysfunction with pulmonary oedema, or display on-going ischaemia evidenced by symptoms or ECG changes. Decisions regarding the exact management strategy in ACS can be complex and a specialist should be involved as early as possible after the first steps in the management of the patient have taken place. The timing of investigations and involvement of the specialist team may be dictated by local protocol. An example of a pathway for the management of suspected ACS is shown in Fig. 1.4.

ST Elevation Myocardial Infarction (STEMI)

The management strategy in STEMI differs from that of NSTEMI and unstable angina in that urgent coronary reperfusion is the treatment of choice. This should be primary Percutaneous Coronary Intervention (PCI) at a designated heart attack centre with round-the-clock cardiac catheterization facilities. In situations when a PCI strategy is not available, primary thrombolysis may be considered (Fig. 1.5).

Eligibility for urgent coronary reperfusion is established by assessing the patient's symptoms and ECG changes as described earlier on (Fig. 1.1). The greatest benefit from reperfusion results if symptoms have been present for less than 12 h although treatment can be initiated if symptoms

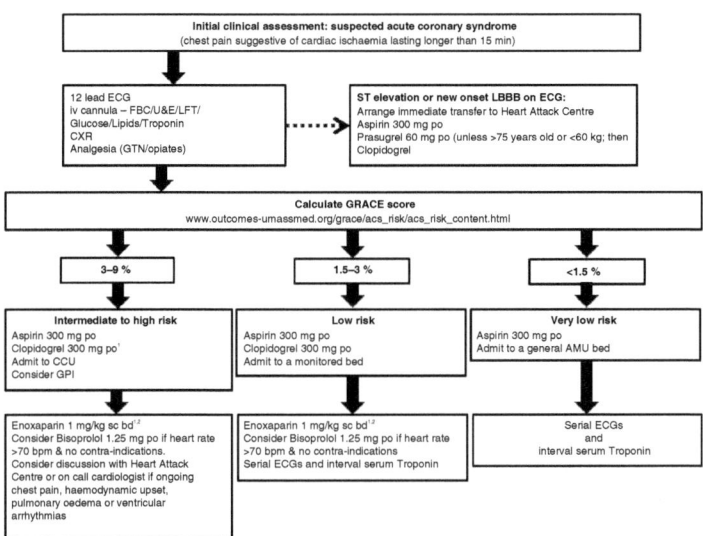

FIGURE 1.4 Local chest pain pathway (Adapted from Royal Shrewsbury and Telford NHS Trust ACS Protocol). [1]Consider deferring if the patient's bleeding risk is unfavourable (e.g. advancing age, female, significant renal impairment or pre-existing anaemia). Refer to crusadebleedingscore.org for more detail. [2]Reduce regime of enoxaparin to OD if age >75 years or eGFR <30

have continued beyond this period if there is ongoing evidence of ischaemia or the pain and ECG changes are stuttering. If primary PCI can be delivered within 120 min of the time when thrombolysis could be administered, the patient should be transferred to a heart attack center for treatment (Fig. 1.5). An initial assessment with regards to the general state of the patient, appropriate analgesia and monitoring should take place in the same way as described earlier for NSTEMI patients. A loading dose of Aspirin 300 mg should be given in all patients but those with a significant allergy. A loading dose of an additional antiplatelet, ticagrelor or prasugrel (the latter if no history of stroke/TIA and age <75) should also be administered. If these newer agents are unavailable, a loading dose of clopidogrel can be used instead.

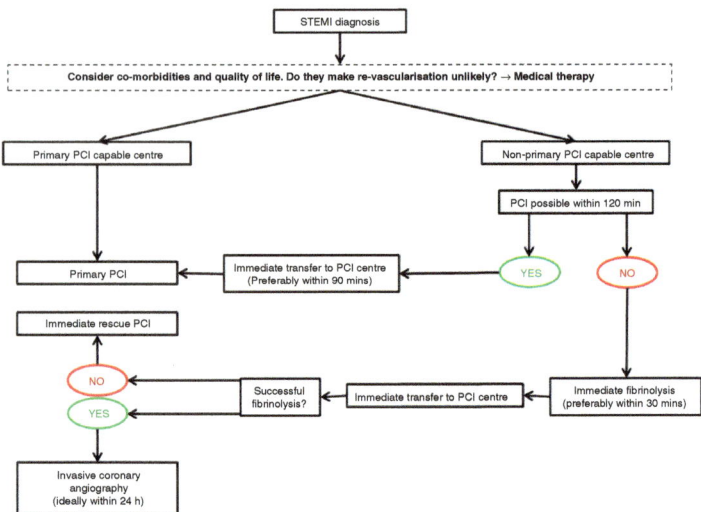

FIGURE 1.5 Reperfusion strategies in patients presenting with STEMI (Adapted from ESC Guidelines for the management of acute myocardial infarction in patients presenting with ST-segment elevation. Eur Heart J. 2012:33;2569–619)

If primary PCI is unavailable or cannot be delivered within 120 min, thrombolysis using an agent such as alteplase, reteplase or tenecteplase may be considered in consultation with a specialist. The potential risks of thrombolysis, in particular that of major haemorrhage or haemorrhagic stroke, should be explained to the patient prior to the drug administration although formal informed consent is not thought to be necessary. The absolute and relative contraindications of thrombolysis are well established and are summarised in Table 1.5.

A patient who has undergone thrombolysis should be monitored continuously for reperfusion arrhythmias. Serial 12 lead ECGs should be performed. Successful thrombolysis is suggested by resolution of symptoms and resolution of the ST segment elevation on the ECG within 60–90 min. In cases of ongoing symptoms and no resolution of the ST segments, a rescue PCI strategy should be contemplated. There is no

TABLE 1.5 Contraindications to thrombolysis

Absolute
Intracranial haemorrhage or stroke with unknown cause
Ischaemic stroke within the last 6 months
Brain tumour or AV malformations
Recent major trauma/surgery/head injury in the last 3 weeks
Known bleeding disorder e.g. haemophilia
Gastrointestinal bleeding within the last month
Aortic dissection
Procedures not amenable to manual haemostasis e.g. liver biopsy within 24 h
Relative
Oral anticoagulant therapy e.g. warfarin
Transient ischaemic attack in the last 6 months
Pregnancy or 1 week post partum
Elevated blood pressure (>180/110 mmHg)
Advanced liver disease
Infective endocarditis
Active peptic ulcer
Prolonged cardiopulmonary resuscitation

evidence to support the use of further thrombolysis in such cases and this should not be considered, as the risk of major bleeding is significant.

Secondary Prevention

A number of pharmacological agents have been shown to confer significant prognostic benefit in patients who are diagnosed with coronary artery disease. In addition to the antiplatelet therapies described above, patients with ACS should be initiated on ACE inhibitors such as Ramipril as soon as they are haemodynamically stable with the dose titrated to the maximum tolerated in a gradual fashion and with monitoring of the patient's renal function.

The long-term use of beta-blockers such as Bisoprolol is now recommended only in patients with left ventricular impairment as guidelines suggest that beta-blockers may be stopped after a year if the LV function is preserved. In practice however, most specialists advocate the long-term use of a beta-blocker in all patients with a history of ACS given their antiarrhythmic properties. In patients with symptoms and signs of left ventricular impairment, the addition the aldosterone antagonist Epleronone is also recommended.

Statin therapy post myocardial infarction is of undoubted benefit and must be considered in all such patients irrespective of the serum cholesterol. Atorvastatin 80 mg is currently recommended but different agents or doses may be considered depending on patient's tolerance and response to therapy.

In addition to pharmacological agents, measures which have been shown to confer profound prognostic benefit in patients treated for ACS include lifestyle changes such as smoking cessation and weight reduction, optimization of blood pressure and diabetic control and exercise based rehabilitation programmes as delivered by multidisciplinary teams.

Stable Angina

Symptom Control

Patients with stable angina will typically describe symptoms on exertion or during periods of emotional stress. A useful classification system is the Canadian Cardiovascular Society (CCS) grading:

Class I: Angina during strenuous or prolonged physical activity

Class II: Slight limitation, with angina only during vigorous physical activity

Class III: Symptoms with everyday living activities, i.e., moderate limitation

Class IV: Inability to perform any activity without angina or angina at rest, i.e., severe limitation

Currently available anti-anginal medications are shown in Table 1.6. These can be effective at relieving symptoms but, with the exception of beta-blockers, there is limited data with regards to any potential prognostic benefit.

A short acting nitrate such as GTN sublingual spray can be used to provide symptomatic relief on an as-required basis. Patients should be given clear instructions with regards to its use during an angina attack and be advised to seek further medical attention if symptoms don't resolve in a timely fashion, usually within 5–10 min. Patients should also be given information with regards to the storage and replenishment of GTN containing formulations over time to ensure easy access to the medication especially when used very infrequently.

Regular anti-anginal medications currently recommended as first line include beta-blockers and calcium channel antagonists which can be combined together for symptom control if necessary. Caution is advised when combining a beta-blocker with a calcium channel blocker given the potential for bradycardias and the use of a dihydropyridine calcium blocker such as Amlodipine is preferred in this instance. If either of these classes of drug cannot be tolerated, other agents that can be used as monotherapy include Nicorandil, Ivabradine, Ranolazine or a long acting oral nitrate. These agents can also be added to a beta-blocker or calcium channel antagonist when symptoms are difficult to control as combination therapy. A third agent may be added if patients remain symptomatic and are not considered suitable for a revascularization strategy (Table 1.6).

Revascularization

The treatment of stable angina by way of coronary artery bypass surgery and PCI may be necessary should medical therapy fail to control symptoms or if there are high risk features on ischaemia testing and risk stratification. Decisions

TABLE 1.6 Anti anginal therapy

Class of drug	Example	Use
Beta blockers	Bisoprolol, metoprolol	1st line
Dihydropyridine calcium channel antagonists	Amlodipine, felodipine	1st line
Non – dihydropyridine calcium channel antagonists	Diltiazem, verapamil	1st line
Nitrates	Isosorbide mononitrate, dinitrate	2nd line
Potassium channel activators	Nicorandil	2nd line
IF channel inhibitors	Ivabradine	2nd line
Late sodium current inhibitors	Ranolozine	2nd line

2nd line agents may used as initial therapy if 1st line agents are not tolerated. If using combination therapy of beta blockers and calcium channel antagonists, avoid non-dihyrdropyridine preparations

with regards to revascularization in stable patients should ideally be made in a multidisciplinary forum involving specialist cardiologists and cardiothoracic surgeons.

Also Worth Knowing

Echocardiography

Echocardiography is recommended for all patients with ACS. It is important to assess ventricular function, so that appropriate therapy can be initiated and to look for the presence or absence of significant valve disease. Patients may be advised to stop driving if the left ventricular function is significantly impaired.

Anaemia

Patients with chronic anaemia are more likely to experience angina symptoms even in the absence of flow limiting coronary artery disease in the epicardial coronary vessels. This is due to the decreased oxygen delivery to the myocardium at a cellular level. Patients with unexplained anaemia should be thoroughly investigated to ensure there is no underlying sinister pathology such as a gastro-intestinal malignancy. Patients with a pre-existing anaemia with a known aetiology should be managed in consultation with a specialist to ensure that their haemoglobin levels remain in the normal range as much as feasible.

Renal Function

Drugs used in the treatment of ischaemic heart disease such as ACE inhibitors and aldosterone antagonists can impair renal function, which should be closely monitored. Contrast induced nephropathy (CIN) following coronary angiography is more likely in patients with pre-existing chronic kidney disease and the risk increases significantly in patients with a low Glomerular Filtration Rate (GFR). Such patients should be managed in consultation with a nephrologist and any planned angiographic procedures are best performed in centers with combined cardiac and renal specialist facilities.

Diabetes

Tight blood glucose control is important in patients with ACS. The aim should be to keep the levels below 11 mmol/l, and this is best achieved with a dose adjusted insulin infusion. Patients who are treated with Metformin should have this discontinued for a period of time around ACS presentation and especially if coronary angiograph is planned as it increases the risk of CIN.

Other Cardiac Conditions Presenting with Chest Pain

Pericarditis

Pericarditis presents as pleuritic central pain, worse on inspiration and lying flat. The patient may have had a recent upper

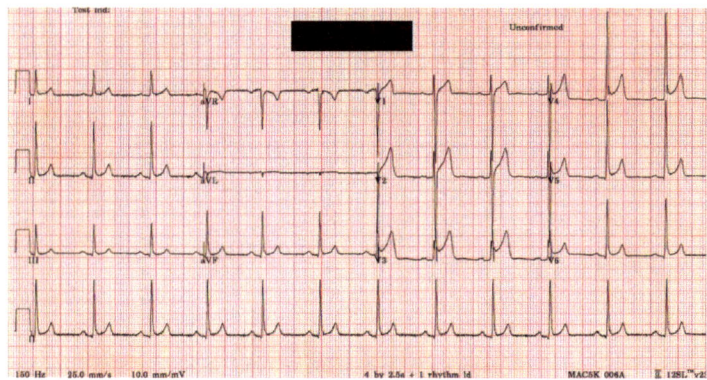

FIGURE 1.6 ECG demonstrating widespread saddle shaped ST segment elevation in a young patient with pericarditis

respiratory tract infection. They may be pyrexial and have raised inflammatory markers.

Clinical examination can be unremarkable but on occasion the patient may have a pericardial friction rub. The ECG shows saddle shaped ST elevation (Fig. 1.6). The echocardiogram is often normal unless there is an associated effusion. There may be an increase in serum troponin levels.

The aetiology may be difficult to diagnose but the commonest causes are:

1. Neoplasia
2. Tuberculosis
3. Autoimmune
4. Viral
5. Purulent (bacterial/fungal)
6. Post myocardial infarction
7. Uraemia
8. Traumatic

Treatment is most effective with non-steroidal anti-inflammatory drugs (ibuprofen, indomethacin, aspirin) or colchicine. Steroids may be indicated in patients with connective tissue disease or refractory pericarditis.

Aortic Dissection

Patients with aortic dissection usually present with severe, tearing anterior or posterior chest pain. Aortic dissection however can present as associated myocardial infarction, stroke, heart failure, cardiac tamponade, paraplegia or other neurological sequelae such as Horner's syndrome.

A history of risk factors such as hypertension, vasculitis, collagen disorders like Marfan's syndrome or a history of congenital heart diseases such as bicuspid aortic valve or coarctation of the aorta should raise the clinical index of suspicion in patients who present with shearing chest pain. The finding of a diastolic murmur of aortic regurgitation or difference in systolic blood pressure of more than 20 mmHg between the two arms in such patients should prompt further investigations. The finding of mediastinal widening on a chest X-ray is not pathognomonic of dissection. A CT aortogram is the investigation of choice in most centers with echocardiography being of some value in unstable patients when dissection of the aortic root is suspected. Patients with aortic dissection should be referred to a cardiothoracic center as an emergency.

Frequently Asked Questions

Q. My patient has had a heart attack, what should I tell them about driving?

A. For group 1 license holders, driving may recommence after 1 week if successfully treated with PCI and no other urgent revascularisation is planned in 4 weeks. The LV ejection fraction must be above 40 %.

If not successfully treated by PCI, driving should cease for 4 weeks. You do not have to inform the DVLA. Further information can be found at www.gov.uk/government/publications/at-a-glance

Q. The patient is on warfarin and is admitted with an NSTEMI, what should I do?

A.   This is always challenging, but the importance of anti-platelet therapy should not be underestimated. Aspirin and a $P2Y_{12}$ inhibitor should be given as advised earlier in the chapter and the warfarin stopped. If the INR is below 2.0, LMWH/fondaparinux should be administered as per guideline/protocol.

Q.   I am concerned about prescribing triple therapy (aspirin/$P2Y_{12}$ inhibitor/warfarin) long term after ACS.

A.   Always discuss this scenario with a cardiologist. Factors to take into consideration include indication for anticoagulation, type of stent used and bleeding risk.

Q.   A surgeon wishes to stop the $P2Y_{12}$ inhibitor for an operation. Is it safe to do so?

A.   It may not be and this will depend on whether the patient has had PCI recently and the type of stent used. Do not stop the medication until it has been discussed with a cardiologist.

Q.   A patient presents to me 72 h after a suspected ACS. How should I manage them?

A.   If the patient has signs of complications such as pulmonary oedema, an urgent assessment in hospital should be organized. If they are completely asymptomatic, take an ECG and troponin level and then make a clinical judgment as to whether the patient should be seen urgently or not.

Q.   I sometimes find it difficult to decide whether a patient's symptoms are consistent with ACS or aortic dissection.

A.   This can be challenging. The clinical history is vital and usually provides you with the information to make a diagnosis. Severe, tearing pain of sudden onset, radiating to the back tends to favor a diagnosis of dissection whereas severe anterior pain of a crescendo nature points more towards an ACS. Use the chest X-ray and blood pressure differentials to help and consult a specialist if still in doubt. Occasionally, imaging the aorta may be the only option.

Red Flags

ST-depression in leads V1-V3 with associated dominant R-wave should raise suspicion suggestive of isolated posterior STEMI.

ST-segment elevation in lead aVR, particularly when associated with precordial lead ST depression is suggestive of left main stem ischaemia.

In STEMI, if primary PCI can be delivered within 120 min of the time when thrombolysis could be administered, the patient should be transferred to a heart attack centre for treatment.

Caution is advised when combining a beta-blocker with a calcium channel blocker given the potential for bradycardias and the use of a dihydropyridine calcium blocker such as Amlodipine is preferred in this instance.

Chapter 2
Dyspnoea: Focus on Heart Failure

Lynne Millar and Sanjay Sharma

Background

The American Thoracic Society defines dyspnoea as 'a term used to characterize a subjective experience of breathing discomfort that is comprised of qualitatively distinct sensations that vary in intensity. The experience derives from interactions among multiple physiological, psychological, social, and environmental factors, and may induce secondary physiological and behavioural responses'. This in-depth definition infers that breathlessness is a complex entity, which can be caused by many conditions. The majority of conditions presenting with breathlessness are respiratory or cardiac in origin (Fig. 2.1). Comprehensive discussion of all of these conditions is beyond the scope of this chapter, which

L. Millar, MB BCh, BAO, MRCP
S. Sharma, BSc(Hons), MBChB, MD, FRCP, FESC (✉)
Cardiovascular Sciences Research Centre,
Cardiovascular and Cell Sciences Research Institute,
St George's University of London, London SW17 0RE, UK
e-mail: lynnemillar@doctors.org.uk; sasharma@sgul.ac.uk

J.C. Kaski et al. (eds.), *Investigating and Managing Common Cardiovascular Conditions*, DOI 10.1007/978-1-4471-6696-2_2,
© Springer-Verlag London 2015

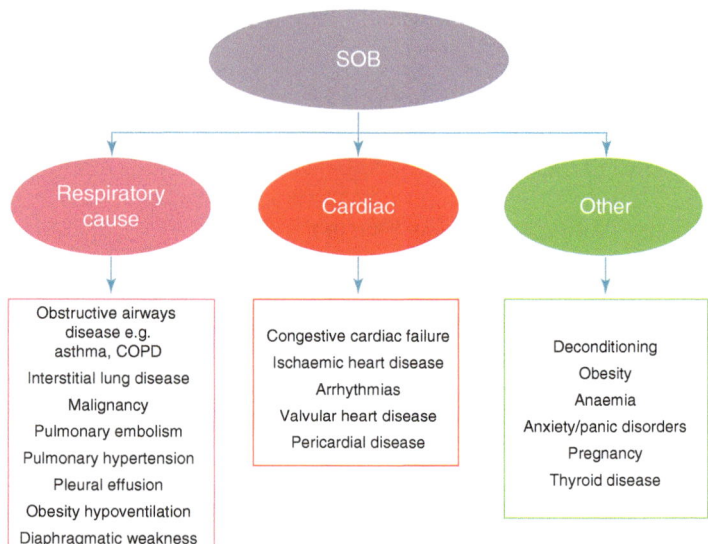

FIGURE 2.1 Differential diagnosis of dyspnoea. *SOB* shortness of breath

negotiates the clinical approach to a patient presenting with breathlessness with a primary focus on the management of chronic heart failure.

Definition of Heart Failure

Heart failure (HF) is a common clinical syndrome whereby the heart fails to meet the metabolic demands of the body. Heart failure represents the end-stage of a number of structural and functional cardiac disorders that impair the ability of the ventricle to fill with (diastolic dysfunction) or eject (systolic dysfunction) blood. The clinical diagnosis of heart failure is based on the presence of a triad of typical symptoms, signs and objective evidence of a structural or functional cardiac abnormality (as assessed by an imaging modality or serum natriuretic peptides). The clinical features of heart failure are attributed predominantly to a reduction in cardiac output (fatigue, weakness) and to increased pulmonary or systemic venous congestion and fluid accumulation (dyspnoea, oedema, hepatic congestion and ascites).

Epidemiology

Heart failure has reached epidemic proportions worldwide, affecting approximately 2–3 % of the world's population. Despite treatment advances within the past few decades patient outcome is still poor, with a 5 year survival <50 %, which represent a survival time that is worse than that for most cancers. The primary causes of death are either progressive pump failure or sudden cardiac death secondary to ventricular arrhythmia. Hospitalisation figures for heart failure are also very high, which places a huge financial burden on healthcare resources.

Causes of Heart Failure

Causes of heart failure are outlined on Table 2.1

Types of Heart Failure

Heart failure can be differentiated into systolic versus diastolic, left versus right and low versus high output heart failure. Most patients will suffer from a low output state due to structural or functional heart disease. Examples of high output heart failure include severe anaemia, thyrotoxicosis and Paget's disease. Right and left heart failure refers to whether the patient has predominantly systemic venous congestion (swollen ankles, hepatomegaly) or pulmonary venous congestion (pulmonary oedema) and do not necessarily reflect which ventricle is affected most.

TABLE 2.1 Causes of heart failure

Ischaemic heart disease	Accounting for 70 % of patients with heart failure in the developed world
Idiopathic	Sporadic Familial in up to 50 % of cases
Valve disease	Accounting for 10 % of patients with heart failure
Hypertension	The primary cause of heart failure in patients of African/Caribbean descent
Alcoholic cardiomyopathy	
Tachycardia-induced cardiomyopathy	Often atrial fibrillation or flutter but any long-standing supraventricular tachycardia High burden of ventricular ectopy/arrhythmias
Other acquired causes	Myocarditis (usually viral, other infectious causes include HIV, Chaga's disease, Lyme disease) Peripartum cardiomyopathy Infiltrative disease (amyloidosis, sarcoidosis, haemochromatosis) With other systemic conditions: thyroid disease, connective tissue disease Stress-induced or Takotsubo cardiomyopathy Iatrogenic (chemotherapy, radiotherapy) Nutritional (Beri-Beri)
Other inherited cardiomyopathies	Arrhythmogenic right ventricular cardiomyopathy Left ventricular non-compaction Burnt out stage of hypertrophic cardiomyopathy

Heart Failure with Preserved Ejection Fraction

Heart failure with preserved ejection fraction, also known as diastolic heart failure refers to abnormal cardiac relaxation or filling. It is characterised by a normal or near normal ejection fraction (usually >50 %) and normal left ventricular end-diastolic volume, with echocardiographic evidence of diastolic dysfunction. It is important to note that impaired diastolic function and diastolic heart failure are not synonymous. As part of the ageing process a number of individuals develop a degree of diastolic dysfunction, but not every one with diastolic dysfunction has diastolic heart failure. The diagnosis of heart failure with preserved ejection fraction or HFpEF requires the presence of symptoms and signs of heart failure. Management of diastolic heart failure primarily requires identifying and treating the underlying cause, however a strong evidence-base is lacking for most of the treatments used currently. General management principles include meticulous blood pressure control, control of ventricular rate in arrhythmias such as atrial fibrillation and use of diuretics for symptomatic relief of fluid overload. Despite the systolic function being preserved, diastolic heart failure is not a benign condition, with diastolic heart failure having a similar prognosis to that of systolic heart failure.

How to Assess Individuals with Dyspnoea

History

A detailed history is important in investigating the cause of breathlessness, as in many cases the diagnosis or a good differential can be gained (Table 2.2). In those with established heart failure it is important to document their New York Heart Association (NYHA) class (Table 2.3), as it provides a measure of their functional capacity and forms the basis for a

TABLE 2.2 Questions you must ask patients presenting with dyspnoea and the potential differential diagnosis

Question	Interpretation
Duration/pattern of breathlessness	This helps determine the chronicity of the condition.
Exercise tolerance	Quantify degree of breathlessness with regards to exercise tolerance using NYHA class.
Symptoms related to reduced cardiac output	Fatigue
Symptoms related to fluid overload	Orthopnoea, breathlessness that is worse on lying flat. Paroxysmal nocturnal dyspnoea Peripheral oedema and ascites Polyphonic wheeze: usually in keeping with obstructive airways disease such as COPD and asthma although can occur in heart failure, so-called 'cardiac asthma'. Sputum: white in keeping with COPD, white-pink usually in keeping with pulmonary oedema, yellow-green usually in keeping with infection or suppurative lung disease.
Gastrointestinal symptoms	Abdominal distension and pain, anorexia, bloating, nausea, constipation and jaundice secondary to congestive hepatomegaly, ascites, reduced bowel perfusion and oedema
Genitourinary symptoms	Oliguria/anuria, urinary frequency, nocturia secondary to impaired renal perfusion
Cerebrovascular symptoms	Confusion, memory impairment, anxiety, headaches, insomnia, bad dreams or nightmares, psychosis with disorientation, delirium, or hallucinations secondary to cerebral hypoperfusion and associated electrolyte abnormalities

TABLE 2.2 (continued)

Question	Interpretation
Musculoskeletal symptoms	Gout, carpal tunnel syndrome, muscle cramps
Past cardiac history	Ischaemic heart disease, hypertension or valvular heart disease are risk factors for heart failure. Cardiac arrhythmias especially atrial fibrillation with a fast ventricular response, can present with breathlessness
Past respiratory history	Do they have established pulmonary pathology such as obstructive airways disease, previous pulmonary embolism, bronchiectasis or pulmonary fibrosis.
Other past medical history	Do they have a known history of diabetes, thyroid disease or HIV? These can be risk factors for heart failure. Do they have a history of allergic rhinitis or atopic eczema? These may predispose to asthma. Any history of bleeding disorders or anaemia? Anaemia itself may cause shortness of breath. Are they deconditioned or obese? Being overweight itself can lead to a subjective feeling of shortness of breath Do they have a history of autoimmune disease or a rheumatological condition? This may predispose them to pulmonary fibrosis. Any history of neuromuscular disorders e.g. motor neurone disease which can lead to respiratory muscle weakness and breathlessness. Any past psychiatric history? As there may be a psychogenic component to the breathlessness.

(continued)

TABLE 2.2 (continued)

Question	Interpretation
Social history	There may be several environmental factors which could predispose or exacerbate symptoms. Smoking history: this could predispose to COPD or ischaemic heart disease or exacerbate asthma. Does the patient have any pets? Pets may predispose to extrinsic allergic alveolitis or asthma. What is the patient's occupation? In certain jobs the patient may be exposed to chemicals or toxins which can cause or aggravate certain conditions. Exposure to carcinogens could lead to lung cancer or asbestos exposure could lead to asbestosis or predispose to lung cancer. Asthma can be exacerbated by several chemicals and therefore is not uncommon among painters, hairdressers and domestic staff. A characteristic feature of this type of asthma is amelioration of the symptoms when away from work or on holiday.
Drug history	Have they started any new medications which could induce breathlessness? Are they on any long term drugs e.g. amiodarone or methotrexate which predispose to lung fibrosis? Have they had previous chemotherapy? Certain chemotherapeutic agents can cause a dilated cardiomyopathy. If they are on long-term pharmacological therapy do they comply with their medications?

number of therapeutic interventions. It is also important to remember that heart failure is a multi-system disorder so patients may present with gastrointestinal, genitourinary and cerebrovascular symptoms.

TABLE 2.3 NYHA Classification of heart failure

Class I	No limitation of physical activity
Class II	Slight limitation of physical activity. Comfortable at rest, but normal daily activities cause breathlessness
Class III	Marked limitation of physical activity. Comfortable at rest, but less than normal activity results in breathlessness
Class IV	Severe limitation. Breathless may be present at rest

Clinical Examination

General Inspection

- It is important to establish the patient's vital signs including blood pressure (to ensure haemodynamic stability and exclude hypertension), oxygen saturations, pulse (rate and whether regular or irregular).
- Is there pallor suggestive of anaemia or cyanosis suggestive of hypoxia?
- Is there nicotine staining on the fingers, suggestive of smoking history?
- Assess for finger clubbing which can occur in lung cancer, suppurative lung disease, congenital cyanotic heart disease and endocarditis.

Cardiovascular System

- Begin by assessing the radial and carotid pulse. Document the rate, rhythm and character.
- Measure the jugular venous pressure (JVP), to check for fluid overload.
- Palpate the apex beat. Is it displaced? Lateral displacement can occur in patients with left ventricular enlargement.
- Are the heart sounds normal and regular? Are there any added sounds for example, a third heart sound (S3) in left ventricular failure or a fourth heart sound (S4) suggestive of a stiffened left ventricle, or murmurs to suggest valvular heart disease.

- Listen for pericardial rub which could be a sign of pericardial inflammation.
- Is there peripheral oedema (pitting), if so how high does it extend? (this may be indicative of right or biventricular failure).

Respiratory System

- Are there abnormalities of the chest wall e.g. a barrel shaped chest which may be in-keeping with longstanding chronic obstructive pulmonary disease (COPD).
- Is chest expansion equal? If it is unequal this could be a sign of pneumonia, pleural effusion or pneumothorax.
- What is the character of the percussion note? A dull percussion note can be suggestive of pneumonia/collapse but a stony dull percussion note is in keeping with a pleural effusion.
- Polyphonic wheeze is usually in keeping with obstructive airway disease such as asthma or COPD but can also be due left ventricular failure (so called 'cardiac asthma').
- Is there bronchial breathing? The presence of bronchial breathing is suggestive of pneumonia but can rarely be caused by localised pulmonary fibrosis or at the air-fluid interface of a pleural effusion.
- Are there any crackles and if so are they coarse or fine? Early inspiratory coarse crackles suggest pneumonia or bronchiectasis whereas both pulmonary fibrosis and pulmonary oedema cause fine inspiratory crackles. Classically pulmonary fibrosis causes late inspiratory crackles whereas pulmonary oedema causes early to mid coarse inspiratory crackles (Table 2.4).

Investigation of Dyspnoea

Bloods Tests

A full blood picture is recommended to check the white cell count (and neutrophil count) which might suggest infection and haemoglobin to exclude anaemia. Anaemia in itself can cause breathlessness, and patients with heart failure and

TABLE 2.4 Examination findings that point towards a diagnosis of heart failure or lung disease

	Heart failure	Pneumonia	Lung fibrosis
Temperature	$\leftrightarrow$	$\leftrightarrow/\uparrow$	$\leftrightarrow$
JVP	$\uparrow$	$\leftrightarrow$	$\leftrightarrow$
Peripheral oedema	Yes	No	No[a]
Chest expansion	Equal	Reduced on affected side	Reduced but equal
Percussion	$\leftrightarrow$ (unless effusions)	dull	$\leftrightarrow$
Crackles	Coarse inspiratory crackles (early/mid)	Coarse inspiratory crackles (unilateral)	Fine end-inspiratory crackles

[a]Unless they develop pulmonary hypertension and cor pulmonale; $\uparrow$ = raised, $\leftrightarrow$ not raised/normal

anaemia (Hb <11 g/dl) generally have poorer outcomes. Measurement of blood chemistry (including sodium, potassium, calcium, urea/blood urea and creatinine/glomerular filtration rate), liver function, thyroid function and iron studies should be performed. These baseline tests are important to detect reversible causes of heart failure e.g. thyroid dysfunction. They are also important to have as a baseline when initiating pharmacological therapies e.g. ACE-inhibitors/aldosterone antagonists. Baseline liver function should be obtained as this may be abnormal in alcoholic cardiomyopathy, α_1 antrypsin deficiency, haemochromatosis and hepatic congestion which can be seen in severe heart failure. C-reactive protein (CRP) can also be done looking for infection.

The use of natriuretic peptides is largely dependent on local resources. They are particularly useful in making the diagnosis in the community. Either beta-natriuretic peptide (BNP) or NT-proBNP can be used. Normal levels have a high negative predictive value making heart failure unlikely as a cause of the patient's breathlessness. Raised levels suggest underlying heart failure (although levels can be raised for other reasons) but very high levels are associated with adverse outcomes and therefore urgent referral to a heart failure specialist is required; the UK National Institute of Clinical Excellence (NICE) suggest within 2 weeks. Natriuretic peptide levels can also be utilised for monitoring in patients with established diagnosis of heart failure as they correlate with morbidity and prognosis.

Electrocardiogram

Electrocardiograms (ECGs) are an important initial step in the work-up of heart failure. Although there are no specific changes related to heart failure, in the vast majority of cases the resting 12 lead ECG exhibits abnormalities and therefore a normal ECG should raise the possibility of an alternative diagnosis for the breathlessness. It is useful to examine the ECG systematically as outlined below:

- What is the heart rate?
  Tachycardia is common in untreated heart failure.
- Is it regular or irregular?
  Cardiac arrhythmias especially atrial fibrillation can themselves cause breathlessness or they may be a manifestation of a secondary pathology such as heart failure.
- Are the QRS voltages normal?
  Voltage criteria for left ventricular hypertrophy may be in keeping with long-standing hypertension, aortic stenosis or less commonly hypertrophic cardiomyopathy.
  Low QRS voltages may be in keeping with infiltrative disease such as Amyloidosis.
- Are there pathological Q waves or T wave inversions?
  These can be suggestive of previous myocardial infarction although non-specific T-wave inversions can be seen with underlying primary cardiomyopathies.
- Are there underlying conduction system defects, for example left bundle branch block or non-specific interventricular conduction delay?
  These findings may be seen in those with previous myocardial infarction, hypertensive heart disease or underlying cardiomyopathy.

TABLE 2.5 Chest X-ray findings to distinguish between heart failure and respiratory causes of breathlessness

Heart failure	Lung pathology
Pulmonary congestion with alveolar oedema	Hyper-expansion of the lung fields (COPD or asthma)
"Bat's wing" shadowing	Reticulo-nodular shadowing (can be localised or diffuse in pulmonary fibrosis)
Upper lobe diversion	Focal consolidation[a] with air-bronchograms[b] (usually pneumonia)
Small effusions: blunting of costo-phrenic angles	Large pleural effusions: uniformly dense white opacification overlying the costro-phrenic angle and hemi-diaphragm with a meniscus
Kerley B lines and pleural effusions (usually small and bilateral)	
Cardiomegaly	

[a]Although consolidation is often used to describe a lobar pneumonia it is not synonymous with it as consolidation can be caused by cancer, pulmonary haemorrhage and pulmonary oedema
[b]In consolidation the small airways fill with dense material (which appear white) however there is relative sparing of the larger airways (these appear darker) which gives the appearance of an air bronchogram

Chest X-ray

Radiographic features suggestive of heart failure are discussed in Table 2.5.

Arterial Blood Gases

When dealing with patients with breathlessness especially in the acute setting baseline blood gas analysis is important. It is important to ascertain if the patient is in type 1 or type 2 respiratory failure. Common causes of type 1 respiratory failure include pulmonary embolism, pleural effusions and congestive cardiac failure whereas type 2 respiratory failure is most commonly seen in patients with exacerbations of COPD. In reality it is rarely that straightforward, as we often see mixed metabolic and respiratory patterns.

Echocardiography

Echocardiography is mandatory for confirming the diagnosis. Apart from documenting systolic and diastolic left ventricular function, the scan is useful in the identification of various causes and complications of heart failure. If an echocardiogram identifies normal cardiac structure and function, despite strong clinical suspicion, consider an alternative diagnosis or referral for a specialist review. Below is a summary of specific features that might be used to ascertain the cause of SOB:

- systolic function: usually documented as a percentage of ejection fraction.
- regional wall motion abnormalities (RWMA) or global systolic impairment. Regional wall motion abnormalities are usually suggestive of ischaemia whereas global impairment suggests a more diffuse cardiomyopathic process
- chamber sizes especially LV dimensions (these are often enlarged in a dilated cardiomyopathy or reduced in size in hypertrophic cardiomyopathy
- diastolic dysfunction: usually documented as mild, moderate or severe (also referred to as grade II-IV diastolic filling patterns)
- valvular pathology: most commonly mitral regurgitation, aortic stenosis
- pulmonary arterial pressures: to assess for pulmonary hypertension (this may co-exist with left ventricular disease, be a consequence of pulmonary pathology or may be present on its own suggesting it is the primary pathology)
- Pericardial disease: due to acute or chronic pericarditis, pericardial constriction, pericardial effusion

- Other pathology: congenital cardiac anomalies such as atrial or ventricular septal defects
- Other complications: intramural thrombus, ventricular aneurysms

Specialist Tests

Cardiac MRI

This modality is complementary to echocardiography. It can be crucial in deciphering the exact aetiology of heart failure especially when a primary cardiomyopathy is suspected. It can give further information about cardiac structure and function. Gadolinium contrast is usually used to look for the presence of late gadolinium enhancement which is suggestive of myocardial fibrosis and scar. The pattern of the late gadolinium enhancement can help distinguish from ischaemic heart failure, myocarditis or an inherited cardiomyopathy.

Coronary Angiography

Coronary angiography may be undertaken in those patients with heart failure of presumed ischaemic aetiology or those in whom the aetiology is unclear.

Cardiopulmonary Exercise Testing

It is widely established that exercise tolerance predicts outcome in patients with heart failure. Cardiopulmonary exercise testing or CPET can be used in heart failure patients as an objective measure of exercise tolerance through measurement of peak VO_2 (maximal oxygen consumption). It can also be used in the context of advance heart failure in risk stratification of patients evaluated for potential heart transplantation.

Other Tests to Consider

Investigations to consider for selected patients with heart failure include

- Blood tests: Troponin I or T, iron studies, folate, vitamin B12, Autoimmune screen, Immunoglobulins and protein electrophresis, serum ACE.
- Viral titres
- Urine sample: Albumin/Creatinine ratio, 24-h urine collection for protein, catecholamines, Bence-Jones protein.
- Pulmonary function tests
- Ambulatory ECG monitoring (Holter)
- Stress imaging
- Radionucleotide ventriculography
- Coronary angiography (CT or conventional)
- Myocardial biopsy
- Right heart catheterisation

Management of Heart Failure (Fig. 2.2)

The initial investigations of choice and the timing of these in patients with presumed heart failure are dependent on the chronicity of the symptoms. In those with an acute presentation, admission to hospital may be the most appropriate step. In patients with a less fulminant presentation they can often be worked up in the community. Caution needs to be taken in patients with a history of ischaemic heart disease, valvular pathology and cardiomyopathies who should be referred for specialist assessment. In most other patients an electrocardiogram and a chest X-ray are performed in the first instance. Depending on the results, a decision is made to proceed to measure serum natriuretic peptides and perform echocardiography (Fig. 2.3). In those with a typical history and investigations suggestive of heart failure, initial pharmacological

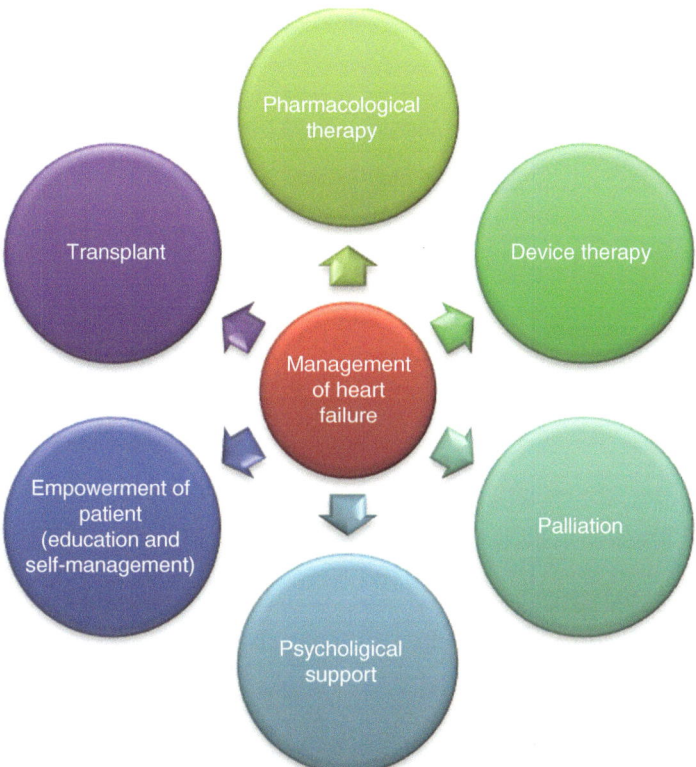

FIGURE 2.2 Overview of the management of heart failure

therapy such as loop diuretics, ACE-inhibitors and β-blockers can be commenced by the primary care physician pending referral to secondary care. Some patients may have the diagnosis and initial management started by their cardiologist or heart failure specialist but are subsequently referred back to the primary care physicians for further management. Community heart failure nurses have an important role in monitoring titration of medications, monitoring weight and fluid balance as well as giving psychological support.

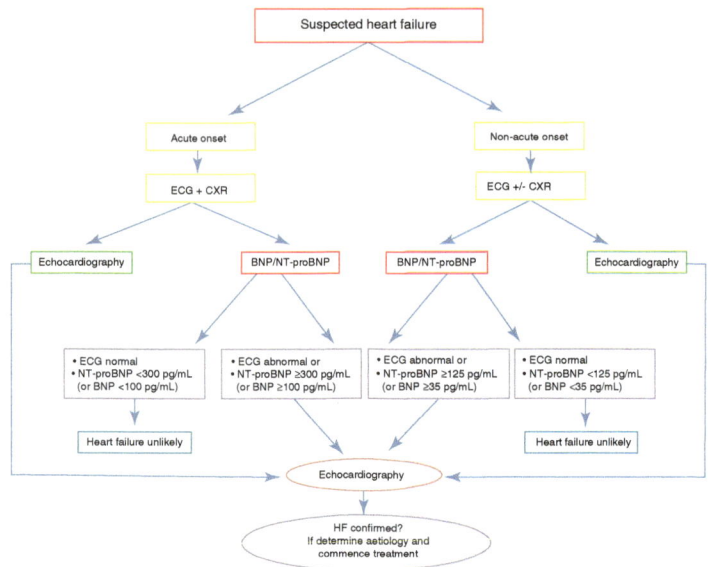

FIGURE 2.3 Algorithm of investigation of suspected heart failure (ESC 2012 Acute and Chronic Heart Failure guidelines – Eur Heart J. 2012;33:1787–847)

Specific Role of the Cardiologist

Patients should be referred to a cardiologist or heart failure specialist in the following settings:

- new diagnosis of heart failure
- patients with NYHA III-IV symptoms
- heart failure due to valve disease
- heart failure refractory to treatment
- those who cannot manage at home
- in women with heart failure who wish to or are pregnant (the care of these patients should be shared between the heart failure specialist and obstetrician)

Patient Education

It is important to educate patients and their relatives in order to empower them to manage their condition in the community and prepare them for the lifelong healthcare interventions required (Fig. 2.2). Table 2.6 outlines all essential topics that should be addressed.

Pharmacological Therapy

Figures 2.3 and 2.4 summarise a treatment algorithm for patients with symptomatic heart failure and reduced systolic function. As a general principle angiotension converting enzyme inhibitors (ACEi), beta-blockers and loop diuretics form the first-line treatment. The mineralocorticoid antagonists or angiotensin receptor blockers are reserved for those who are still symptomatic despite optimal first-line treatment or who cannot tolerate one or more of those agents. Other pharmacological agents and device therapy is reserved for patients with persistent symptoms or patients with specific characteristics as described below.

Loop Diuretics

Loop diuretics provide symptomatic relief from pulmonary and systemic congestion by reducing fluid overload, however, they do not offer any prognostic benefit. Regular monitoring of renal function and electrolytes is required to avoid renal failure, hyponatraemia, hypokalaemia and hypomagnesaemia. It is important to start with a low dose, especially in diuretic-naive patients and the elderly, and increase the dose until clinical improvement occurs. Once fluid overload resolves the diuretic dose should be readjusted to avoid dehydration. Motivated patients should be educated about

TABLE 2.6 Education topics that should be addressed in patients with heart failure

Educational topics	Skills and self-care behaviours
Education of the condition and the cause	Explain to patients what the condition is and why they have the symptoms they have.
Symptoms and signs of heart failure	Empower patients so they can recognize signs and symptoms of decompensation. Allow the patient flexibility in adjusting their diuretic dose.
Pharmacological treatment	Understand indications, dosing and effects of drugs. Recognise the common side-effects of each drug.
Risk factor modification	Counsel the patient regarding smoking cessation. Monitor blood pressure if hypertensive. Ensure good blood glucose control if diabetic.
Diet recommendation	Salt restriction. Avoid excessive fluid intake. Modest intake of alcohol Monitor and prevent malnutrition
Exercise recommendation	Be reassured, comfortable about physical activity Understand the benefits of exercise.
Sexual activity	Discuss problems with healthcare professionals. Be reassured about engaging in sex and understand specific sexual problems and various coping strategies.
Immunization	Receive immunization against infections such as influenza and pneumococcal disease

TABLE 2.6 (continued)

Educational topics	Skills and self-care behaviours
Compliance	Understand the importance of following treatment recommendations Maintaining motivation to follow treatment plan
Psychosocial aspects	Understand that depressive symptoms and cognitive dysfunction are common in patients with heart failure and the importance of social support Learn about treatment options if appropriate
Prognosis	Understand important prognostic factors and make realistic decisions. Seek psychosocial support if appropriate

self-adjustment of their diuretic dose based on daily weight measurements and other clinical signs of fluid retention.

Angiotension Converting Enzyme Inhibitors (ACEi)

Unless contraindicated or not tolerated, all patients with symptomatic heart failure or asymptomatic left ventricular dysfunction should receive an ACEi. Angiotension converting enzyme inhibitors reduce morbidity (improve symptoms, exercise tolerance, quality of life and reduce the need for hospitalisation) and mortality and may improve or at least prevent further deterioration of ventricular function. The main concern relating to ACE-inhibitors is deterioration in renal function and hyperkalaemia. This may or may not be in the presence of renal artery stenosis. Some rise in urea and creatinine (up to 10 %) is expected and should not cause concern. An increase of ≤ 50 % from baseline or to an absolute concentration of 265 µmol/l, whichever is lower, is acceptable. If creatinine rises to >265 µmol/l but is <310 µmol/l,

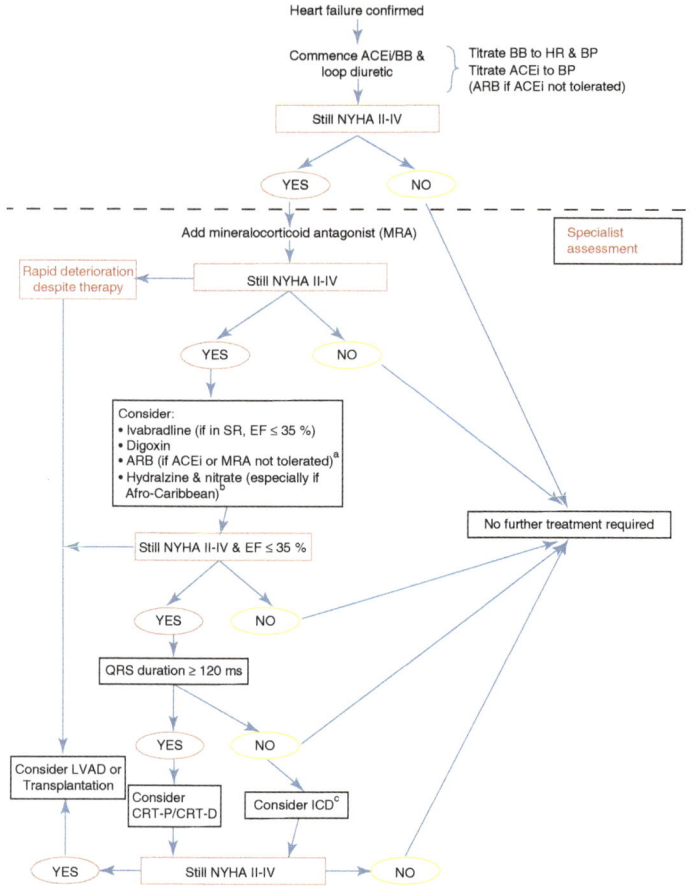

FIGURE 2.4 Algorithm to the management of heart failure (Adapted from ESC 2012 Acute and Chronic Heart Failure guidelines – Eur Heart J. 2012;33:1787–1847). [a]If mineralocorticoid receptor antagonist not tolerated, an ARB may be added to an ACE inhibitor as an alternative. [b]The combination of hydralazine and isosorbide dinitrate may also be considered earlier in patients unable to tolerate an ACE inhibitor or an ARB. [c]ICD is not indicated for NYHA IV. Asymptomatic patients with an LVEF ≤35 % and a history of myocardial infarction should be considered for an ICD

halve the dose of ACEi and monitor biochemistry. If creatinine rises to ≥310 μmol/l, stop ACEi and monitor biochemistry. In case of hyperkalaemia, if potassium rises to >5.5 mmol/l, halve the dose of ACEi and monitor biochemistry. If however the potassium rises to >6.0 mmol/l, stop the ACEi and review. Ensure that the patient is not on any other nephrotoxic drugs or drugs that could exacerbate hyperkalaemia.

A potentially life threatening side effect is the development of angioedema, but that occurs in only 0.1–0.7 % of individuals and usually resolves on discontinuation. Finally, dry cough and hypotension may limit the drug's utility.

Contraindications to ACEi

- history of angioedema
- bilateral renal artery stenosis
- serum creatinine >220 μmol/l
- severe aortic valve stenosis

Initiation of ACEi

Below is a simple guide on how to initiate and titrate ACEi

- check renal function and serum electrolytes.
- start with a low dose and re-check renal function and serum electrolytes within 1–2 weeks of commencing the treatment.
- consider dose up-titration at 2–4 week intervals and re-check renal function and serum electrolytes within 1–2 weeks of dose up-titration.
- more rapid dose up-titration can be carried out but close supervision is required.
- once maintenance dose has been achieved re-check renal function and serum electrolytes at 1, 3, 6 months and 6 monthly thereafter.
- aim for evidence-based target dose or the maximum tolerated dose (in practical terms this is highest dose that BP will allow).

Angiotensin II Receptor Blockers

Angiotensin II receptor blockers (ARBs) should be used in patients with heart failure or asymptomatic left ventricular systolic dysfunction when an ACE-inhibitor is not tolerated (usually due to cough). As with ACE-inhibitors, ARBs reduce morbidity and mortality in these patients. Currently the addition of an ARB on top of optimal ACE-inhibitor treatment should be considered in heart failure patients who remain symptomatic despite optimal doses of ACE-inhibitor and β-blocker, when aldosterone antagonists are either not tolerated or contraindicated.

Contraindications and Initiation Protocol

As with ACE-inhibitors.

Beta-Blockers

Unless contraindicated or not tolerated all patients with symptomatic heart failure or asymptomatic left ventricular dysfunction should receive a β-blocker. Beta-blockers reduce morbidity (improve symptoms, exercise tolerance, quality of life and reduce the need for hospitalisation) and mortality, and may improve or at least prevent further deterioration of ventricular function. Beta -blockers should be initiated as soon as possible when a diagnosis of heart failure is made; however it is wise to wait at least 24 h when someone has presented in pulmonary oedema as this therapy can initially worsen heart failure symptoms. Beta-blockers should be titrated to heart rate, aiming for a heart rate of 50–60. Compared to ACE-inhibitors they have a minimal effect on blood pressure but in those patients with SBP < 100 mmHg caution needs to be taken. In contrast to popular belief, chronic obstructive pulmonary disease is not a contraindication to the use of β-blockers. Lung function tests with assessment for reversible airways obstruction may prove a useful adjunct. If significant reversibility exists re-evaluate the COPD diagnosis and perform a trial with a short acting β-blocker. Asthma is also not an absolute contraindication. In severe cases, beta-blockade is best avoided but in less severe cases small doses can be tried under a specialist's supervision. For example, a low dose of short acting β-blocker such as Metoprolol 12.5 mg could be given, and oxygen saturation and PEFR could be monitored before and after. If there are significant asthmatic symptoms induced or reduction in the PEFR beta-blockers should be avoided. Finally, β-blockers should be used with extreme caution is patients with significant bradycardia, particularly in the presence of high degree heart block or sick sinus syndrome.

Main Side-Effects

- Fatigue: can be a direct side effect of β-blockers not related to bradycardia or hypotension.
- Bradycardia: Perform an ECG and/or ambulatory monitoring to exclude significant heart block or pauses. If heart rate is <50 beats per minute and the patient is symptomatic discontinue other contributing drugs prior to reducing, or as a last resort, stop the β-blocker dose and monitor the patient.
- Erectile dysfunction: This is often under-reported. When reviewing patients it is important to ask about these sensitive issues as patients may be too embarrassed to bring it up. Reducing the beta-blocker dose may improve symptoms. Consider referring for a specialist opinion or the use of phosphodiesterase inhibitors. Caution should be taken in those with co-existent hypotension or nitrate use.

Mineralocorticoid Receptor Antagonists

Mineralocorticoid receptor antagonists (MRAs) are the only diuretics that have been shown to improve outcome (reduced mortality and hospital admissions) in patients with heart failure. Evidence from large trials has shown benefit of spironolactone and eplerenone. Eplerenone is indicated in a specific sub-group of post-acute myocardial patients with LVEF ≤40 % and heart failure or diabetes (EPHESUS trial) or in those developing endocrine side effects on Spironolactone (10 % of males may develop breast tenderness or enlargement).

The main concern relating to MRAs is deterioration in renal function and hyperkalaemia. If the creatinine rises to >210 μmol/L, halve the dose and monitor biochemistry. If however, the creatinine rises to ≥310 μmol/L, stop the MRA and monitor biochemistry closely. As with ACEi, if potassium rises to >5.5 mmol/l, halve the dose of the MRA and if it rises to >6.0 mmol/l, discontinue it and monitor biochemistry.

Contraindications

- serum potassium >5.0 mmol/l
- serum creatinine >220 μmol/L
- addition to a combination of ACE-inhibitor and angiotensin receptor blocker

Initiation of Aldosterone Antagonists

- check renal function and serum electrolytes.
- re-check renal function and serum electrolytes 1 and 4 weeks after starting treatment.
- consider dose up-titration after 4–8 weeks. Do not increase dose if worsening renal function or hyperkalaemia. Re-check renal function and serum electrolytes 1 and 4 weeks after increasing dose.
- aim for evidence-based target dose or maximum tolerated dose.
- re-check renal function and serum electrolytes 1, 2, 3, and 6 months after achieving maintenance dose, and 6 monthly thereafter.

Cardiac Glycosides (Digoxin)

Digoxin is a useful aid to β-blockers for rate control of atrial fibrillation in patients with heart failure but its role is less well established in patients with sinus rhythm or rate controlled atrial fibrillation. Data from trials has shown that it improves symptoms, quality of life and reduces hospitalisations due to heart failure but it has not shown to reduce mortality. It can be used prior to the initiation of a β-blocker in patients with decompensated heart failure and should be considered where β-blockers are contraindicated. Furthermore digoxin should be considered in symptomatic patients on optimal medical treatment i.e. on ACE-inhibitor, β-blocker and aldosterone antagonist irrespective of the need for heart rate control. In the majority of patients, oral dosing (rather than intravenous) is appropriate.

Contraindications

Digoxin should be avoided in those in patients with significant bradycardia (<50 beats per minute) or high degree heart block and in patients with evidence of accessory pathway on their ECG.

Common Side-Effects

- Conduction abnormalities, gastrointestinal upset, blurring or yellow haloes in visual field.
- Toxicity can occur, especially in patients with renal failure therefore therapeutic monitoring is important. Additionally hypokalaemia and drugs such as Amiodarone and certain antibiotics can increase the risk of toxicity.

Hydralazine and Isosorbide Dinitrate

In chronic heart failure the combination of Hydralazine and Isosorbide dinitrate should be considered as an alternative to an ACEi or ARB in patients who do not tolerate either of these drugs, or as an addition to patients on optimal medical therapy i.e. ACEi/ARB + β-blocker + MRA, who remain symptomatic. Patients of African or African-Caribbean descent, seem to benefit to a greater extend from the use of this combination (A-HeFT trial). Initiation should be at a dose of Hydralazine 25 mg three times daily and ISDN 20 mg three times daily, aiming for a target dose of Hydralazine 75 mg and ISDN 40 mg three times daily. Monitoring for drug-induced lupus is required. The combination should be avoided in individuals who exhibit symptomatic hypotension, severe renal impairment or have a diagnosis of systemic lupus erethymatosous (SLE).

Ivabradine

Ivabradine should be considered in patients with stable heart failure, who are in sinus rhythm and despite maximally tolerated beta-blocker their heart rate remains ≥70 bpm. Unlike beta-blockers ivabradine works on the I_f sodium channel in the sino-atrial node. It does not affect blood pressure and therefore it can be better tolerated in patients with relative hypotension. On a practical note, this drug should only be commenced around a month after being already established on conventional heart failure therapy, by a heart failure specialist. The starting dose is 5 mg twice daily aiming to titrate to 7.5 mg twice daily in 2 weeks. Reduce ivabradine to 2.5 mg twice daily if the heart rate drops below 50 bpm. This may be the preferred starting dose in frail elderly patients. The main side effects of this medication are symptomatic bradycardia but this should be observed for in the weeks after initiation. Other side effects include visual disturbances and dizziness.

Device Therapy

Cardiac resynchronisation therapy (CRT), is also known as biventricular pacing as the device paces simultaneously the right and the left ventricle. The rationale behind this therapy is that in patients with bundle branch block on their ECG there is dyssynchronous contraction of the two ventricles and restoring interventricular synchrony improves cardiac efficiency. CRT has been shown to improve symptoms, reduce hospitalisations and prolong survival in patients with symptomatic heart failure and severe systolic impairment, who are in sinus rhythm. Evidence for benefit from CRT in individuals with persistent or permanent AF is not as strong as in sinus rhythm, though the predominant predictor of improved outcome is the percentage of successful biventricular pacing. Since ventricular rates are frequently fast, conducted intrinsic beats may lead to failure to pace. Therefore, in patients with <99 % biventricular pacing, ablation of the AV junction to render patients pacing dependent may be appropriate.

Two main types of therapy exist: a biventricular pacemaker with pacing function alone, known as a CRT-P (P standing for pacemaker) and a biventricular pacemaker with a defibrillation function, known as a CRT-D (D standing for defibrillator with additional anti-tachycardia therapies). Some patients do not meet the criteria for resynchronisation therapy but may be a candidate for an implantable cardioverter defibrillator (ICD), alone.

Indications for ICD as Primary Prevention in Heart Failure

- LVEF ≤35 %
- NYHA II-III
- on optimal medical therapy ≥3 months
- expected to survive more than a year
- If ischaemic aetiology, at least 40 days post acute myocardial infarction

Indications for CRT-P

- LVEF ≤35 %
- NYHA II-IV symptoms
- QRS duration ≥120 ms with LBBB or QRS duration ≥150 ms with other conduction delay

In order for someone to be a candidate for CRT-D they need to fulfil both criteria.

Telemonitoring

Over the past few years telemonitoring has been set up to facilitate early discharge of patients from hospital and reduce heart failure related admissions. It requires a multidisciplinary team approach, integrating hospital and community heart failure teams. The evidence is unclear as to whether it truly incurs benefit but it is probable that it will become more commonplace in the future due to stretched inpatient heart failure resources.

Transplant

In patients with rapidly deteriorating heart failure or in those with deterioration despite optimal medical therapy, it may be appropriate to consider cardiac transplantation. When contemplating a referral to a transplant centre it is important to be realistic with the patients, as many will not be suitable candidates or may die on the transplant list due to donor shortage. Due to the shortage of donor hearts strict criteria are in place as to who should receive a transplant (Table 2.7). Left ventricular assist devices (LVADs) are mechanical devices which augment or partially replace the circulatory function in the failing heart. In the UK and the rest of Europe they are mostly used as a bridge to transplantation but in the future they may be considered as destination therapy in their own right.

Palliative Care

In those with advanced heart failure, whose symptoms are resistant despite aggressive medical or device therapy, palliation should be considered. Symptomatic relief may be the most appropriate management strategy. A multidisciplinary team approach should be adopted involving the patient, their family, the heart failure nurses, cardiologists and the palliative care team. End stage heart failure can be extremely traumatic for both patients and their families. Good communication between all parties is imperative to ensure that the

TABLE 2.7 Indications and contraindications to transplantation

Patients to consider cardiac transplantation
End-stage heart failure despite maximal therapy
Motivated patient, well informed & emotionally stable
Able to comply with intensive treatment post-operatively

Contra-indications to transplantation
Active infection
Severe PVD or cerebrovascular disease
Current alcohol or drug abuse
Treated for cancer within the past 5 years
Unhealed peptic ulcer
Recent thrombo-embolism
Significant liver disease
Systemic disease with multiorgan involvement
Other serious co-morbidity with poor prognosis
Psychiatric illness/emotional instability
High pulmonary vascular resistance (>4–5 Woods units and mean transpulmonary gradient >15 mmHg)

patient's spiritual, religious, psychological needs are addressed and the patient remains as comfortable as possible. This may be co-ordinated through the palliative care team who have expertise in dealing with patients at the end of life. Patients with ICDs should be counselled and it should be ensured the ICD function is turned off.

Common Problems/Comorbidities Associated with Heart Failure

In light of the patient demographics and aetiology for heart failure, significant comorbidities may be encountered in these patients.

Anaemia

Patients with anaemia and heart failure have a higher morbidity and mortality. Anaemia in these patients is likely to be multifactorial i.e. renal impairment, dilutional effect, inflammatory response that affects the bone marrow. A standard diagnostic work-up should be undertaken in anaemic patients and all correctable causes should be treated. Correction of iron deficiency with Intravenous iron therapy should be considered. The value of erythropoietin-stimulating agents as a treatment for anaemia of unknown aetiology in heart failure patients remains of uncertain benefit.

Depression

Depression is common among patients with heart failure and it is associated with poor outcomes. Of importance, depression is associated with poor compliance with heart failure therapy. A high index of suspicion is required to recognise and treat early. Serotonin selective reuptake inhibitors are the drug of choice, while tricyclic antidepressants should be avoided as they may cause hypotension and exacerbate heart failure symptoms.

Kidney Dysfunction

It is well established that patients with renal impairment have a much poorer outcome in heart failure. Although minor reductions in glomerular filtration rate are seen in patients who are commenced on ACEi and ARBs, dramatic and continuing reductions should raise suspicion of renal artery stenosis. Aldosterone antagonists should be used with caution in patients with renal impairment and patients should be carefully monitored for hyperkalaemia especially if used in conjunction with ACEi.

Erectile Dysfunction

Erectile dysfunction is not an uncommon side effect in heart failure patients. It may be due to the co-existence of diabetes or use of β-blockers. Phosphodiesteradse inhibitors can be used but should be avoided in patients on nitrates and caution should be exercised in patients with hypotension.

Obstructive Airways Disease

It is not uncommon for patients with heart failure symptoms to have coexisting obstructive airways disease. Patients may not be clear of the exact diagnosis and may report a history of asthma when in fact they have COPD. It is important to establish the correct diagnosis as physicians are often reluctant to prescribe β-blockers in individuals with a past medical history of asthma. Furthermore, the coexistence of these conditions makes the assessment of heart failure patient's challenging as it is often difficult to differentiate the cause of the patient's symptoms.

Gout

Hyperuricaemia and gout are common in heart failure and may be caused or aggravated by diuretic treatment. Hyperuricaemia is an independent risk factor of poor prognosis. Acute attacks should be treated with colchicine rather than NSAIDs. Intra-articular corticosteroids are an alternative for monoarticular gout. Xanthine oxidase inhibitors such as allopurinol may be used to prevent gout.

Diabetes Mellitus

Tight glycaemic control is recommended. Thiazolinediones have been associated with increased fluid overload and symptomatic heart failure and are therefore contraindicated. Given the close association of heart failure and renal dysfunction, renal function should be monitored in patients on Metformin, which may require discontinuation in acute exacerbations associated with acute on chronic renal failure.

Body Weight

Being over or under-weight is associated with poorer outcomes in patients with heart failure. Cachexia is associated with more symptoms, reduced functional status, more hospitalisations and reduced survival. The diagnosis of heart failure in obese patients can be challenging. In part the breathlessness that they experience is due to deconditioning and body habitus. Moreover, confirming the diagnosis in obese patients through echocardiography can be difficult due to poor echocardiographic windows.

Frequently Asked Questions

How quickly should I up-titrate a patient's ACE-inhibitor and beta-blocker?

In the outpatient setting it is appropriate to up-titrate ACE-inhibitors and β-blockers at 2–4 weekly intervals (however this could be more aggressive if the patient is strictly monitored). Generally speaking ACE-inhibitors can be titrated to systolic blood pressure of 90–100 mmHg providing the patient is not symptomatic whereas beta-blockers are titrated to a target heart rate of 50–60 bpm again providing the patient is asymptomatic. In the inpatient setting these medications can be titrated much more aggressively but β-blockers should be omitted for the first 24 h in those presenting with acute pulmonary oedema. See also relevant section under ACEi.

When is it appropriate to add in an MRA?

Providing the patient meets the appropriate criteria (see section on MRA) and once the patient is on the maximum tolerated beta-blocker and ACEi an MRA can be introduced. In patients presenting with acute myocardial infarction, Eplerenone is indicated early on (3–14 days post event) in the presence of systolic left ventricular dysfunction and heart failure (EPHESUS trial), irrespective of whether optimal ACEi and beta-blocker doses have been achieved. This therapy is usually initiated by a cardiologist or heart failure specialist in secondary care.

My patient has asthma/COPD, do I have to adjust their medication?

This question is often asked and many patients are denied beta-blockers due to concerns over exacerbating their COPD (see relevant section under beta-blockers). In the first instance it is important to establish what the diagnosis is and what was it based on. If in doubt, lung function tests with assessment for reversible airways obstruction may be useful.

Most patients with COPD and mild to moderate severity asthma can tolerate cardioselective beta-blockers well. If in doubt, small doses of short acting beta-blockers such as Metoprolol can be tried under a specialist's supervision.

Must Do's

- check 12 lead ECG, if normal re-evaluate the diagnosis
- treat reversible causes
- establish baseline renal function and monitor renal function after each dose adjustment
- titrate drugs to the maximal tolerated dose
- think about transplantation early in young patients and those with rapid deterioration despite optimal medical therapy

- educate the patient about their condition, their medications and the importance of compliance
- ensure the patient has the appropriate support and/or put them in contact with the heart failure nurses.

Red Flags

- Think of heart failure in patients with persistent cough and SOB that does not respond to conventional therapy, usually comprised of antibiotics and bronchodilators.
- Patients with multiple hospital admissions should be managed by a heart failure specialist team.
- Young patients presenting with severe systolic dysfunction should be considered early for evaluation in a transplant centre.
- Dilated cardiomyopathy with associated conductive tissue disease and malignant family history, think of Lamin A/C gene mutation.

Also Worth Knowing

Acute Decompensation in Heart Failure

Acute pulmonary oedema is managed with intravenous loop diuretics and vasodilators such as glyceryl trinaitrate (GTN) or Morphine. Recent evidence suggests that patients with acute pulmonary oedema have a much better prognosis when admitted to highly monitored acute beds under a specialist, such as a coronary care unit, and therefore if this is feasible it is best to do so. Further treatment options include the use of Continuous Positive Airway Pressure (CPAP) which can aid diffusion and can help drive fluid back into the capillary beds from the alveolar spaces. In some centres haemofiltration is utilised to relieve severe fluid overload, although its efficacy over and above large dose diuretics has not been conclusively established. If, despite these measures, the patient continues to deteriorate, admission to the intensive care unit may be necessary for inotropic and/or mechanical support in addition to invasive ventilation. Once the patient is stable, it is imperative to identify the cause for acute decompensation.

Causes of Acute Decompensation

Non-cardiac

- Non-compliance with medication or life-style advice (very common and may be due to lack of patient education)
- Concomitant infection e.g. chest sepsis
- Anaemia
- Alcohol
- Other drugs (non-steroidals)

Cardiac

- Arrhythmias (commonly AF)
- Ischaemia
- Worsening valve disease
- Bradyarrhythmias

Heart Failure in Pregnancy

Heart failure in pregnancy can be due to an exacerbation of pre-existent heart failure or development of peripartum cardiomyopathy. Peripartum cardiomyopathy is defined as heart failure developing in the last month of pregnancy or within 5 months of delivery, in the absence of another identifiable cause. The aetiology is unknown. One hypothesis is that it is a type of idiopathic dilated cardiomyopathy which is unmasked by the physiological stresses of pregnancy. Another theory is that it is due to the effects of prolactin on the heart and therefore bromocriptine (which blocks the release of prolactin from the pituitary gland) is sometimes used to treat it. Due to the complexity of heart failure in pregnancy, a multidisciplinary team approach should be applied with input from cardiologists, heart failure specialist and the obstetricians. Pharmacological therapy can be challenging in pregnancy and in lactating women. Beta-blockers are generally safe in pregnancy and although are excreted in the breast milk, they are generally safe during breast-feeding. For those with fluid overload, simple loop diuretics can be used. Angiotension Converting Enzyme inhibitors are contraindicated in pregnancy, but in selected cases they may be commenced by a specialist. For those requiring vasodilation antepartum, hydralazine is the drug of choice as anecdotal evidence suggests it is safe in this setting. For those who cannot tolerate hydralazine, amlodipine is a suitable alternative. In some women with rapid deterioration in their clinical state, delivery is the safest option and the risks and benefits of breast feeding need to be addressed. Prognosis is variable with some women having full recovery of their cardiac function whereas others are left with residual heart failure. Sensitive issues like contraception and the safety of further pregnancies should be addressed.

Further Reading

ESC Guidelines for the diagnosis and treatment of acute and chronic heart failure 2012. Eur Heart J. 2012;33:1787–847.
2013 ESC guidelines on cardiac pacing and cardiac resynchronization therapy. Eur Heart J. 2013;34:2281–329.

Online Resources from the National Institute for Health and Care Excellence (NICE)

http://pathways.nice.org.uk/pathways/chronic-heart-failure
http://pathways.nice.org.uk/pathways/acute-heart-failure

Chapter 3
Palpitations

Anthony Li and Magdi M. Saba

Introduction

The term "palpitations" refers to the sensation of an abnormally perceived heart beat. This common symptom is a frequent reason for referral to the cardiology clinic and can be the cause of considerable anxiety in some patients. Conversely, a high incidence of anxiety disorders is also seen in this group of patients. A significant proportion of patients may not have a detectable arrhythmia following extensive investigation. However, identifying the minority of patients who have a clinically significant arrhythmia is important. Some arrhythmias carry the potential to be life-threatening; others can be

A. Li, MBBS, MRCP
Cardiovascular Sciences Research Centre,
Cardiovascular and Cell Sciences Research Institute,
St George's University of London,
London SW17 0RE, UK
e-mail: anthonyli@doctors.org.uk

M.M. Saba, MD, FHRS (✉)
Cardiac Electrophysiology, St. George's Hospital
and University of London, London, UK
e-mail: msaba@sgul.ac.uk

J.C. Kaski et al. (eds.), *Investigating and Managing Common* 67
Cardiovascular Conditions, DOI 10.1007/978-1-4471-6696-2_3,
© Springer-Verlag London 2015

readily treated for symptomatic relief. Correct identification of these diagnoses is clearly critical.

This chapter aims to provide an overview of the management of patients with palpitations, with a focus on the most common arrhythmia, atrial fibrillation (AF).

Differential Diagnosis

The differential diagnosis of palpitations is broad and can be classified according to perceived rhythm and rate (Fig. 3.1). Beyond this, a 12 lead electrocardiogram (ECG) of the rhythm captured whilst symptoms were present is essential to make a firm diagnosis. However, a carefully taken history can be suggestive of a diagnosis.

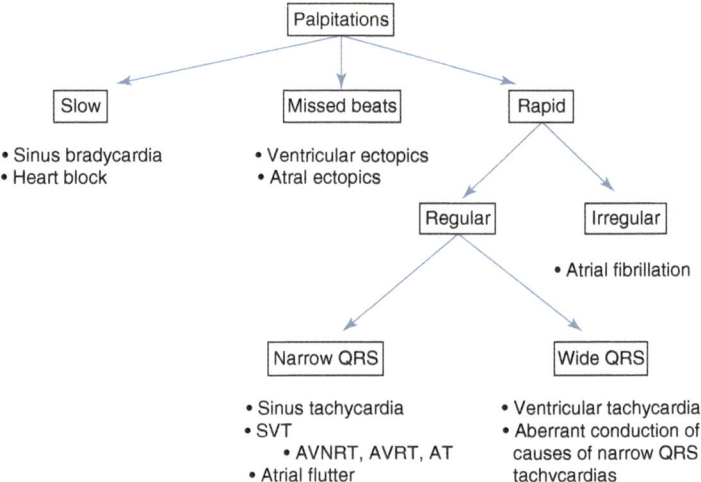

FIGURE 3.1 Classification of palpitations according to history and ECG findings. *Abbreviations*: *SVT* supraventricular tachycardia, *AVNRT* atrioventricular nodal reentry tachycardia, *AVRT* atrioventricular reentry tachycardia, *AT* atrial tachycardia

General Patient Approach

Patients presenting with palpitations are commonly asymptomatic at the time of presentation. In this case, the focus should be on determining the severity of associated symptoms with a particular emphasis on red flag symptoms, the likely presence or absence of structural heart disease and common reversible causes of arrhythmia. Palpitations in individuals without evidence of structural or functional heart disease generally carry a benign prognosis, except in the rare inherited primary arrhythmia syndromes, such as the long QT and Brugada syndromes.

History

Symptoms

Arrhythmias can manifest with a wide variety of associated symptoms. However, the uncovering of certain "red flag" symptoms or features should prompt referral to a specialist, as they may point to a potentially serious cause (Table 3.1).

Important clues gained from the history may suggest a specific underlying arrhythmia. Ectopic beats are described commonly as pauses ("skipped beats") followed by a more forceful heartbeat. Irregularity may indicate AF or atrial

TABLE 3.1 Red flags

Palpitations with syncope/pre-syncope

Palpitations that worsen with exercise

Family history of inherited heart disease or premature unexplained sudden death

High risk structural or functional heart disease

e.g. myocardial infarction, congenital heart disease, cardiomyopathy flutter with variable conduction, though frequent ectopy can also be described in this way. Abrupt onset and offset of palpitations commonly occur in pathological supraventricular tachycardias (SVT), as opposed to gradual onset and offset associated with sinus tachycardia. Furthermore, polyuria following termination of palpitations may also point towards SVT; polyuria results from natriuretic peptide release in response to atrial stretch. Reliable termination of palpitations with atrioventricular (AV) node blockade (pharmacological or physiological) is highly suggestive of common forms of SVT. Thus, patients may report that vagal manoeuvres such as coughing or Valsalva resolve symptoms. A history of palpitations since childhood may also indicate that SVT involving an accessory pathway (atrioventricular re-entry tachycardia; AVRT) could be the mechanism. Conversely, atrial arrhythmias occur more often in older patients.

Medical History and Examination

Clues from a patient's medical history may also point toward certain forms of arrhythmia. A history of pulmonary disease increases the likelihood of atrial tachycardia (AT). Similarly, mitral valve disease predisposes to AF. A history of possible myocardial scarring, such as prior myocardial infarction or cardiomyopathy should be sought, as their presence in the context of syncope is ominous and points to possible life-threatening ventricular arrhythmias requiring urgent evaluation by a cardiologist.

A multitude of medications may precipitate arrhythmia. Common classes of medications that trigger or exacerbate arrhythmias are the beta agonists, thyroxine and theophyllines amongst others. Over the counter medications such as cough/cold medicines, decongestants and nutritional supplements containing stimulants such as caffeine or guarana can similarly precipitate arrhythmias. Illicit use of amphetamines and cocaine should also be elicited. Alcohol overconsumption should be viewed as a precipitant for AF.

A careful family history is important to identify a potentially inheritable condition. A history of sudden unexplained death under the age of 45 years may indicate heritable cardiac causes such as hypertrophic cardiomyopathy or ion-channel disorders such as the long QT syndrome, Brugada syndrome and catecholaminergic polymorphic ventricular tachycardia (CPVT).

Most patients who present with symptoms of arrhythmia are asymptomatic during the consultation and physical examination is often unrevealing. However, abnormal heart sounds or signs of heart failure indicate the presence of structural heart disease, which predisposes to the development of AF and ventricular tachycardia (VT).

Investigations

Baseline investigations should involve full blood count, electrolytes and thyroid function to exclude anaemia, electrolyte abnormalities and thyroid dysfunction.

A 12-lead ECG should be taken even when asymptomatic at the time of acquisition as it may reveal clues as to the presence of underlying heart disease. As ECG abnormalities may be subtle, it is recommended that the ECG be interpreted by people with the necessary expertise; abnormalities to be scrutinised for are listed in Table 3.2.

In the event that the patient presents with tachycardia, and providing it is not causing severe symptoms and/or haemodynamic instability, an ECG during tachycardia is essential for diagnosis. If the patient experiences sustained palpitations but they are infrequent, then they should be given a covering letter and instructed to attend the local casualty department for an ECG during tachycardia.

Ambulatory monitoring is of use where symptoms are frequent enough to be captured. Frequency of symptoms determine the device to be selected with most hospitals offering 24 h continuous monitoring which is appropriate for patients with palpitations more that 2–3 times in a week and

TABLE 3.2 ECG abnormalities during sinus rhythm

Abnormality	Possible cause
Short PR interval and delta wave	WPW – AVRT
Q waves	Prior MI – VT/AF
P mitrale	Enlarged LA – AF
Prolonged QT interval	Long QT syndrome – VF
ST shift / T wave inversion	HCM – VT/AF
	ARVC – VT/AF
	Prior MI – VT/AF

Abbreviations: *WPW* Wolff-Parkinson-White, *MI* myocardial infarction, *LA* left atrium, *VF* ventricular fibrillation, *HCM* hypertrophic cardiomyopathy, *ARVC* arrhythmogenic right ventricular cardiomyopathy

patient activated 7 day loop recorders for those with less frequent symptoms. Monitoring during asymptomatic periods provides limited information and may also lead to false reassurance. Conversely, normal sinus rhythm captured at the time of symptoms can be reassuring.

When to Refer

A suggested criterion for admission of patients presenting with and without symptoms at the time of consultation is shown in Table 3.3 and Fig. 3.2.

Management of Specific Arrhythmias

Atrial Fibrillation

Atrial fibrillation is the most common sustained arrhythmia worldwide with an estimated prevalence of 1–2 % and is on the rise. It is diagnosed with an ECG demonstrating an irregular RR interval and no distinct P waves (Fig. 3.3). The presence of

TABLE 3.3 Criteria for emergency admission for patients currently experiencing arrhythmia

Any broad complex tachycardia

Persistent narrow complex tachycardia despite vagal manoeuvres

Breathlessness/Chest pain/Syncope/Presyncope

Hypotension

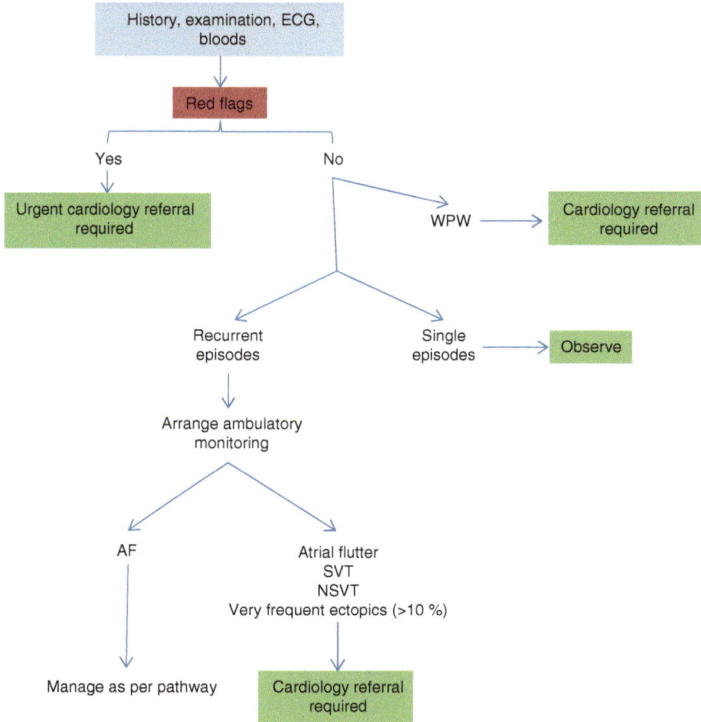

FIGURE 3.2 Referral pathway for patients who are asymptomatic at presentation. *Abbreviations*: *WPW* Wolff-Parkinson-White, *AF* atrial fibrillation, *SVT* supraventricular tachycardia, *NSVT* non-sustained ventricular tachycardia

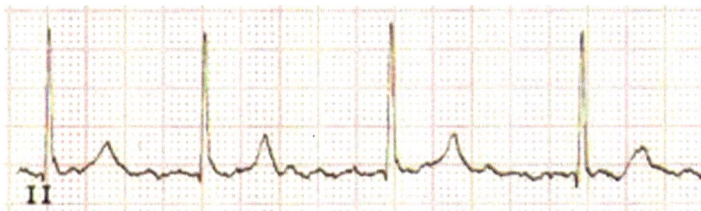

FIGURE 3.3 ECG demonstrating AF with irregular QRS complexes and indiscernible P waves

AF is an independent risk factor for increased mortality and morbidity and carries an approximate 5 fold increased risk of stroke, hospitalisation and 3 fold risk of heart failure. AF is traditionally classified as paroxysmal if duration of episodes is <7 days, persistent if >7 days duration and permanent (or chronic persistent) if it is accepted in the long term.

Over the last few years, the management of AF has evolved considerably with the availability of the novel oral anticoagulants (NOAC) and the increasing role of interventions such as ablation.

The goals of AF management are:

1. Assessment of stroke risk and antithrombotic therapy.
2. Treatment of symptoms with rate or rhythm control
3. Treatment of underlying disease processes.

Stroke Risk Assessment and Anticoagulation

Screening

Screening of individuals aged over 65 years by pulse palpation followed by routine ECG in those who have irregularity should be undertaken to prevent complications of AF before they develop.

Stroke Risk Assessment

Anticoagulation therapy in AF is the only treatment that has been firmly shown in multiple trials to reduce stroke risk.

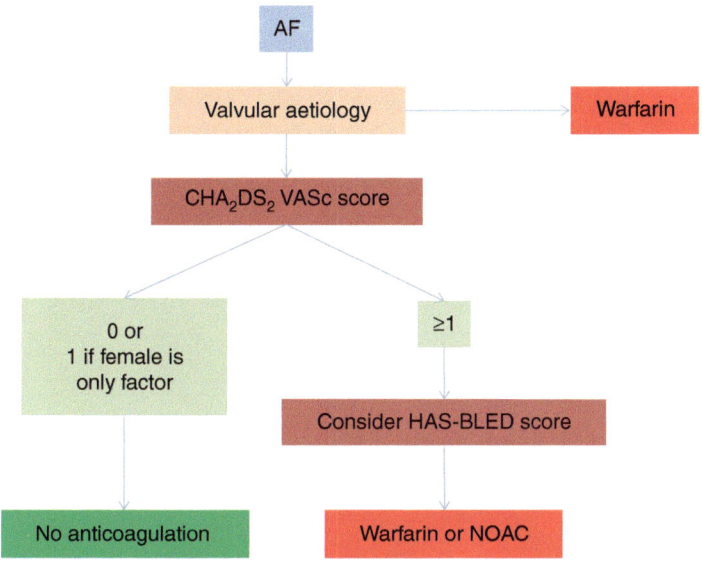

FIGURE 3.4 Anticoagulation decision algorithm – adapted from 2012 ESC guidelines

Furthermore, when evaluating the need for anticoagulation, the risk of stroke should be considered the same regardless of the pattern or frequency of AF.

Several guidelines have been published on stroke risk stratification of AF from different international organisations since 2006, with the emphasis shifting from identifying those at risk of stroke to establishing those who are truly low risk who do not require antithrombotic treatment. This has been formalised in the CHA_2DS_2VASc risk score (Fig. 3.4). This approach was driven by data on newer risk factors that showed that those who were classified previously as being low risk by prior risk-stratification scores (including the commonly applied more-limited $CHADS_2$ score) were still at moderate risk and would benefit from anticoagulation. Furthermore, data on the efficacy of aspirin, which has long been thought of as an alternative to warfarin, is unconvincing, particularly in the elderly and has been shown to have similar bleeding risks to that of warfarin. As a result, the role of

TABLE 3.4 Green denotes low risk – anticoagulation not needed. Red denotes high risk – anticoagulation recommended

CHA$_2$DS$_2$–VASc Score	Adjusted stroke rate (%/yr)
0	0
1	1.3
2	2.2
3	3.2
4	4.0
5	6.7
6	9.8
7	9.6
8	12.5
9	15.2

aspirin has been downgraded and should only be considered where the patient has declined warfarin or a NOAC; unequivocally low-risk individuals require neither antiplatelet nor anticoagulant (Tables 3.4 and 3.5).

Bleeding Risk Assessment

It has been shown that despite the superiority of oral anticoagulation in preventing strokes, studies have consistently demonstrated its underuse in high-risk patients and a high rate of discontinuation. Reasons for this are several fold and include age, fall risk and bleeding risk, which tend to be overestimated by physicians. The HAS-BLED score has recently been developed to provide a more objective bleeding risk assessment and identifies potentially correctable risk factors

TABLE 3.5 CHA$_2$DS$_2$ – VASc Score calculation

Cardiac failure	1
Hypertension	1
Age >75 years	2
Diabetes	1
Stroke/TIA	2
Vascular disease (MI, PVD, aortic plaque)	1
Age 65–74	1
Sex **C**ategory female	1

TABLE 3.6 HAS-BLED Score calculation

Feature	Score
Hypertension (Systolic >160 mmHg)	1
Abnormal renal or liver function	1 or 2
Stroke	1
Bleeding history or predisposition (anaemia)	1
Labile INR (therapeutic time in range <60 %)	1
Elderly ≥65 years	1
Drugs (antiplatelets, NSAIDs) or alcohol excess	1 or 2

(Table 3.6). In patients with a score of ≥3, caution should be exercised and regular review undertaken, but should not be used in isolation to exclude patients from anticoagulant therapy.

Antithrombotic Therapy

The choice of agents for thromboprophylaxis has rapidly expanded in the last few years and novel oral anticoagulants (NOAC) and antiplatelet agents have been extensively investigated in large randomized trials. However, the costs of the newer NOAC may – at least initially – restrict their use to defined groups of patients, despite their efficacy.

As stated previously, the evidence for aspirin in stroke prevention is weak and the risks of major bleeding and intracranial haemorrhage should be considered similar to warfarin, particularly in the elderly. Furthermore, there is no evidence that aspirin reduces cardiovascular mortality in the AF population. The addition of clopidogrel to aspirin is superior to aspirin alone, however with the disadvantage of a greater bleeding risk than warfarin. Warfarin has been the gold standard for many years, with a reduction in risk of stroke by 64 % overall with a major bleeding rate of 3.6 % per year and risk of intracranial haemorrhage of 0.7 % per year. However, its disadvantages include the need for regular blood tests in view of its variability in metabolism. As such, it has been shown that even in the most rigorously conducted trials, patients receiving "optimal" warfarin management were within therapeutic range for only 63 % of the time and is likely to be considerably less in a community setting.

The NOACs dabigatran (Pradaxa), rivaroxaban (Xarelto) and apixaban (Eliquist) have recently been approved for use in the UK by NICE. A comparison of each agent can be seen in Table 3.7. So far, there have been no head to head trials of one NOAC against another, so comparisons on efficacy cannot be made. Currently, robust data exists only for their use in non-valvular AF and there is sparse data beyond this.

In general, the NOACs afford better stroke risk reduction compared with warfarin, mainly due to the reduction in haemorrhagic stroke. In addition, they do not need regular monitoring and have less food and drug interactions. Despite these advantages, the NOACs have several disadvantages when compared with warfarin (Table 3.8).

Concerns have been raised over the current lack of antidotes to the NOACs and the lack of a measure of anticoagulant effect which may become relevant in an emergency setting such as when a patient requires emergency surgery, though the shorter half-life means that urgent surgery can safely take place 48–72 h following the last dose. On the other

TABLE 3.7 Oral anticoagulant options for stroke prevention in atrial fibrillation

	Warfarin	Dabigatran	Rivaroxaban	Apixaban
Dosing	Variable OD	110/150 mg BD	20 mg OD	2.5–5 mg BD
Monitoring	Regular INR with does adjustment	Not needed	Not needed	Not needed
Major bleeding risk vs. warfarin	N/A	Similar at 150 mg Lower risk at 100 mg Increased risk of GI bleeding	Similar to Warfarin overall Increased risk of GI bleeding	Lower than warfarin
Risk of ICH vs. warfarin	N/A	Lower than warfarin	Lower than warfarin	Lower than warfarin

(continued)

TABLE 3.7 (continued)

	Warfarin	Dabigatran	Rivaroxaban	Apixaban
Common side effects	Bleeding related	Bleeding related: anaemia, epistaxis, GI haemorrhage, haematuria. diarrhoea, dyspepsia, nausea	Bleeding related: epistaxis, anaemia, conjunctival haemorrhage, GI haemorrhage. Peripheral oedema, dizziness, nasopharyngitis, dyspepsia, nausea, diarrhoea	Bleeding related: anaemia, epistaxis, contusion, conjunctival haemorrhage
Renal metabolism	Not affected	Avoid in severe renal impairment. eGFR <30 ml/min	Avoid in severe renal impairment. eGFR < 15 ml/min	Avoid in severe renal impairment. eGFR < 15 ml/min

Abbreviations: ICH intracranial haemorrhage, *GI* gastrointestinal, *GFR* glomerular filtration rate

TABLE 3.8 Novel oral anticoagulants

Advantages	Disadvantages
Rapid onset of action	No clinical antidote
Shorter half-life	Missed doses more significant
No need for monitoring	No ability to monitor effect
Less food/drug interactions	Renal impairment increases anticoagulant effect

hand, this may disadvantage patients with poor compliance, since missed doses may leave patients at risk of stroke compared to warfarin, particularly in those that require twice daily administration. In addition, the lack of requirement to attend anticoagulation clinics may further reduce compliance and removes an opportunity for patients to raise issues regarding their care. Evolving renal or hepatic impairment may also pose a risk of increased bleeding to patients on NOACs as they all, to some extent, rely on these routes for excretion and without a method of reliably measuring anticoagulation effect, significant bleeding may occur.

FAQs: Anticoagulation

My patient is currently on warfarin with a stable INR, should I switch them to a NOAC?

Patients should be counselled fully in order to make an informed decision with regards to NOACs. Due to their high cost, availability may be limited to specific indications. Guidance on prescribing NOACs may be produced by local health services for this reason. Example of such guidance include limited use of NOACs to a second line therapy where:

1. A patient is allergic or intolerant of warfarin
2. INR on warfarin is labile and out of therapeutic range for a significant period of time where there is good compliance
3. There are significant problems with access to monitoring INR

How often should I follow up patients on NOACs?

The European Society of Cardiology (ESC) guidelines recommend follow up by the initiator of anticoagulant treatment which can be in primary or secondary care or in dedicated anticoagulation clinics, preferably every 3 months to document adherence, monitor side effects and potential bleeding complications as well as a review of drugs to prevent adverse interactions.

What blood tests are required?

Current guidelines recommend annual full blood count, renal and hepatic function testing. In cases of renal impairment with a creatinine clearance of 30–60 ml/min, monitoring every 6 months is required. In cases where the creatinine clearance is less than 30 ml/min, monitoring every 3 months is recommended. In vulnerable groups such as those >75 years on dabigatran, renal function should be checked every 6 months.

What do I do if my patient is undergoing a planned minor procedure?

For procedures with a minor bleeding risk such as dental extractions and where adequate local haemostasis is achievable, patients with normal renal function should stop the NOAC 18–24 h prior to the procedure. Providing the procedure is uncomplicated, dosing can resume 6 h post-procedure.

First Presentation in Primary Care

If a patient presents for the first time with pulse irregularity and a 12-lead ECG confirms definite AF with no other significant abnormality then the course of action depends on symptoms and duration of AF (Fig. 3.5). In general, if the onset of AF can be identified with certainty to be less than 48 h duration, then admission for cardioversion is reasonable as the risk of thromboembolism becomes higher after this period and the ability to maintain sinus rhythm after successful cardioversion decreases. However, due to poor symptom-arrhythmia correlation in AF, it is more frequently the case that the onset is unclear. If the patient is highly symptomatic or has signs of

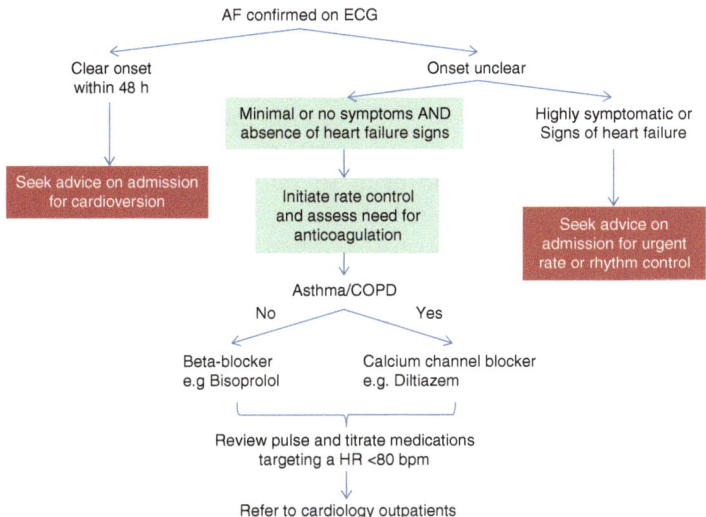

FIGURE 3.5 Management algorithm for first presentation of atrial fibrillation (AF) confirmed on ECG to clinic

heart failure then admission for urgent rate control is needed. If the patient currently in AF has minimal or no attributable symptoms or heart failure signs, then assessment of stroke risk followed by initiation of rate control with either beta-blocker or calcium channel blocker is reasonable. Patients should then be reviewed for titration of medication doses to achieve a resting heart rate of 80 bpm. If further rate control is required, the addition of digoxin may be required. Digoxin may also be a reasonable first choice drug in the less active, elderly AF population but should not be first line in other groups as its efficacy is limited during exercise.

Role of the Cardiologist

The role of the cardiologist is to counsel patients on rate versus rhythm control strategies and the various treatment options available for each, in order to achieve optimal symptom control and deal with complex issues related to anticoagulation. Part of the evaluation should also involve the assessment of underlying structural heart disease and other complications of AF (e.g. tachycardia induced cardiomyopathy), as this will inform subsequent strategy and influence the type of antiarrhythmic drug to be given. Monitoring for adverse effects of antiarrhythmics should be shared between primary and secondary care. AF ablation is a rapidly expanding area and patients may be deemed suitable for this approach at an early stage.

Rate Versus Rhythm Control

The decision to adopt a rate or rhythm control strategy has been influenced by the lack of effective and safe antiarrhythmic therapy. Two of the largest trials (AFFIRM and AF-CHF) that sought to answer the question of which strategy is best failed to find a survival benefit of either strategy. This lack of benefit was thought by many to be due to the adverse effects and lack of efficacy to maintain sinus rhythm of the currently available antiarrhythmic agents.

The current ESC guidelines suggest an individualised approach. In general, the decision is based on how adequately symptoms are controlled after rate control has been initiated. It is also informed by a judgement on how likely it is that sinus rhythm is able to be maintained, the type of AF and underlying disease processes contributing to the perpetuation of AF. Although evidence is sparse, there is increasing recognition that there may be a window of opportunity to intervene before the transition from paroxysmal to persistent/permanent AF occurs. This transition is thought to indicate irreversible electrical and structural remodelling of the atria, which significantly reduces the success of rhythm control strategies, including ablation. In rare circumstances, where antiarrhythmic drugs are contraindicated or ineffective and AF ablation is unsuitable, AF may be controlled by ablation of the AV node and permanent pacemaker therapy.

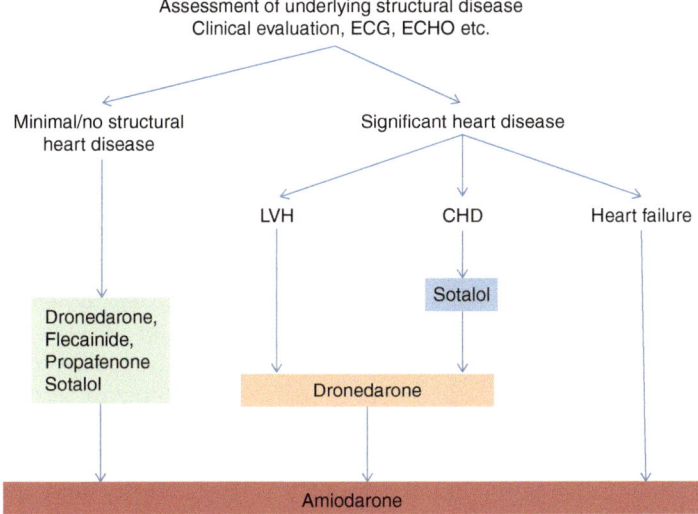

FIGURE 3.6 Algorithm for prescription of antiarrhythmic drugs for the treatment of AF according to absence or presence of heart disease. *Abbreviations*: *LVH* left ventricular hypertrophy, *CHD* coronary heart disease (Adapted from 2012 ESC guidelines on the management of AF)

Rhythm Control

Antiarrhythmic Drugs

Antiarrhythmic drugs are generally used as long-term therapy, however in carefully selected patient groups, a "pill in the pocket" approach may be warranted for those with infrequent, highly symptomatic episodes, who have been counselled adequately.

The choice of antiarrhythmic drug is dictated by the presence or absence of structural heart disease (Fig. 3.6). In general, antiarrhythmic drugs are moderately effective (50–60 % success) for maintaining sinus rhythm at 12 months. In a large meta-analysis, antiarrhythmic drugs as a group reduced the recurrence of AF in the region of 30–55 % in patients after cardioversion. Head to head comparisons between drugs is lacking but amiodarone has been shown to be the most effective. It is also considered safe in the setting of structural heart disease, with a low pro-arrhythmic risk, but has significant adverse effects leading to discontinuation in up to 70 % at 5 years. For this reason, amiodarone should reserved for when other therapies have failed or are contraindicated. Before commencing amiodarone, patients should be counselled on its common adverse effects including, amongst others, corneal opacities, photosensitivity, skin discolouration and tremor. Serious events include hypo/hyperthyroidism in 4 %, pulmonary toxicity including acute pneumonitis and fibrosis in 2 % and abnormalities in liver function in 1 %. Six-monthly blood count, electrolytes, liver and thyroid function testing should be monitored during long-term use. Baseline respiratory evaluation either by pulmonary function testing and/or chest x-ray and annual review with chest x-ray and eye examination are recommended by some, though often only performed in the context of altered symptoms.

Dronedarone (Multaq) is similar in structure to Amiodarone but does not possess the iodine moiety that causes the thyroid, neurological, ocular or dermatological side effects. It is currently unclear what the potential pulmonary or liver toxicity may be and therefore regular monitoring is still warranted. Large clinical trials have shown that it is inferior to amiodarone in maintaining sinus rhythm and, more importantly, have shown that it may cause harm in patients with heart failure and those with permanent AF. This has lead to subsequent revision of international guidelines, restricting its use in these patients.

In addition to extra-cardiac side effects, the other commonly used anti-arrhythmic drugs for AF carry a small but definite pro-arrhythmic risk. Slowing of conduction, as in the case of Class I sodium channel blockers (e.g. flecainide), or delayed repolarization, as in the case of class III drugs (e.g. sotalol), are the basic mechanisms of pro-arrhythmia. With all antiarrhythmic drugs, it is necessary to monitor the QRS duration and QT interval after initiation. In this regard, it is worth specific mention that, while an effective antiarrhythmic second only to amiodarone in long term maintenance of sinus rhythm, sotalol is associated with a risk of QT prolongation and torsades de pointes. As such it should be initiated at a smaller dose, and an ECG performed within 2–3 days of any dose escalation. Monitoring of renal function and electrolytes is also necessary as the risk of pro-arrhythmia increases, particularly with flecainide and sotalol as they are renally excreted.

Cardioversion

Cardioversion of AF can be achieved either electrically or chemically using a variety of agents that are typically used for chronic rhythm control but at higher doses. In carefully selected patients, cardioversion to sinus rhythm can provide relief from highly symptomatic AF and can be performed safely, providing the onset of AF is within 48 h, or anticoagulation within the therapeutic range has been achieved continuously for 1 month beforehand, or transoesophageal echocardiography has ruled out atrial thrombus. In general, cardioversion is more successful the sooner it is attempted after AF onset. Furthermore, it should be considered in the context of a more comprehensive management plan as without the use of additional antiarrhythmic drugs to help maintain sinus rhythm, over half of patients will revert to AF at 1 year. Occasionally, it is also used to evaluate symptomatic benefit from being in sinus rhythm in those who may be considered for ablation.

Catheter Ablation of AF

In 1998, it was discovered that most episodes of AF are initiated by ectopic beats arising from muscle sleeves lining the pulmonary veins entering the left atrium. This knowledge led to the development of minimally invasive percutaneous techniques to electrically isolate the pulmonary veins by applying either radiofrequency, cryothermal or laser energy to create discrete scar lines that eliminate the initiation or prevent

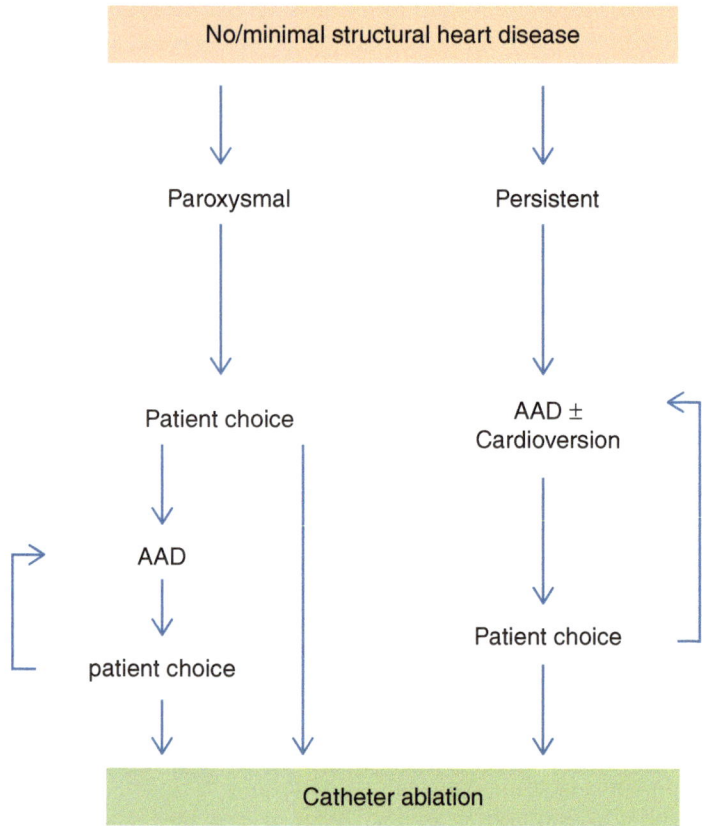

FIGURE 3.7 Algorithm for catheter ablation in atrial fibrillation. *Abbreviations*: *AAD* antiarrhythmic drugs

propagation of AF. In recent guidelines, the indication for catheter ablation has been expanded and may be suitable as first line therapy in carefully selected patients (Fig. 3.7). Catheter ablation can be performed under general anaesthesia or conscious sedation with access to the heart achieved via the femoral veins. The left atrium is accessed by puncturing the inter-atrial septum and the catheters are manoeuvred with the aid of fluoroscopy or by mapping systems that are able to accurately track the tip of the catheter in space to create a 3D model of the atrium. Recent developments include robotic and magnetic navigation systems, which allow the operator to perform the procedure remotely. AF ablation procedures typically last between 2–3 h. Data from recently published trials indicate that catheter ablation of paroxsysmal AF is successful in approximately 50 to >70 % of patients with a single procedure (depending on the technique used) and, when used as a first line therapy, is superior to antiarrhythmic therapy in terms of quality of life and freedom from symptomatic AF at 2 year follow up. In reported trials, patients needed a mean of 1.5 procedures to achieve complete success. However, there is less certainty regarding long-term outcomes from ablation due to rapidly evolving techniques studied and continuously updated catheter technology. Results of on-going large outcome trials are also pending which will report on the efficacy of ablation for morbidity and mortality in due course. Whilst effective, ablation of AF carries a risk of major complications including stroke (0.6 %), cardiac tamponade (1.3 %) and vascular access complications (1.3 %). Patients undergoing cryoballoon ablation are also at risk of phrenic nerve injury (4.7 %) but this is reversible in the vast majority of cases. Patients should therefore be counselled on the risks of ablation, which need to be weighed against individual symptomatic relief.

Ablation of persistent AF is a more challenging procedure with likely reduced success rates after a single procedure. This is thought to be due to atrial remodelling resulting in a change in the underlying mechanism of AF such that structural changes (substrate) within the atria are more able to sustain AF. This has resulted in the development of substrate modification strategies as well as targeted ablation of non-pulmonary vein triggers during ablation that invariably requires more extensive ablation within the atria and the increased likelihood of requiring a repeat procedure to achieve success. Nonetheless, ablation of persistent AF can still provide significant symptomatic benefit compared to antiarrhythmic drug therapy in selected patients.

FAQs: Rate and Rhythm Control

What monitoring is required for patients on amiodarone?

1. Baseline full blood count, electrolytes, Liver function test and Thyroid function then 6 monthly testing thereafter.
2. Baseline respiratory evaluation with chest x-ray and/or pulmonary function testing
3. Yearly clinical respiratory evaluation. Further tests only if development or progression of symptoms e.g. persistent cough or breathlessness
4. Yearly ECG monitoring to check for QT prolongation

What ECG parameters need monitoring in patients taking antiarrhythmic drugs?

QT interval and QRS duration can be derived from automated ECG analysis, which on the whole is reasonably reliable. Automated reports on absolute QT interval and also corrected QT interval (QTc) are provided. The QTc is the value corrected for heart rate and should be used for interpretation.

Initiation of antiarrhythmic therapy should always be accompanied by monitoring of QRS duration, QT interval and for symptomatic bradycardia. If the QTc approaches or exceeds 500 ms or the QRS duration exceeds 120 % of baseline then the therapy should be immediately stopped and urgent advice sought.

Does having a catheter ablation for AF mean that my patient can come off antiarrhythmics?

Following ablation, patients may remain on their antiarrhythmics for upto 3 months for the scar induced by the ablation to form. After this period, antiarrhythmic therapy may be withdrawn in most cases.

Does having a catheter ablation for AF mean that my patient can come off anticoagulation?

All patients are recommended to receive anticoagulation for 2–3 months post ablation. There is currently a lack of data on the long-term recurrence rates of AF post ablation and the effect of ablation on stroke risk. Therefore, patients are assessed by conventional risk scores and anticoagulation continued indefinitely according to their stroke risk and not on the presence or type of AF. Mounting observational evidence suggests a reduction in stroke risk post-ablation in those who maintain sinus rhythm, but no randomized, controlled data exist to date. In exceptional circumstances, where discontinuation of anticoagulation is being considered despite a high stroke risk then patients should undergo a period of continuous monitoring to detect asymptomatic episodes of AF at regular intervals.

My patient is still experiencing palpitations after the ablation, has it worked?

It is common for patients to experience palpitations after the procedure, which may be due to ectopic beats or even recurrent AF or other atrial arrhythmias in the first 3 months as the scar created by ablation takes time to mature and inflammation settles.

Atrial Flutter

Atrial flutter is a re-entrant rhythm that arises from circuits that occupy large areas of either atrium. The most common type involves the right atrium that utilizes a circuit around the tricuspid annulus that typically has an atrial rate of 300 bpm with a ventricular rate of 150 bpm due to 2:1 conduction through the AV node but can vary depending on the ratio of atrial to ventricular conduction. This can produce the appearance of a sawtooth baseline that is more easily seen during higher ratios of atrial to ventricular conduction or after adenosine administration (Fig. 3.8).

The management of atrial flutter is similar in some respects to that of AF including recommendations for anticoagulation, antiarrhythmic therapy and cardioversion. However, there are a few important differences in management to that of AF. In contrast to AF, which is a chaotic

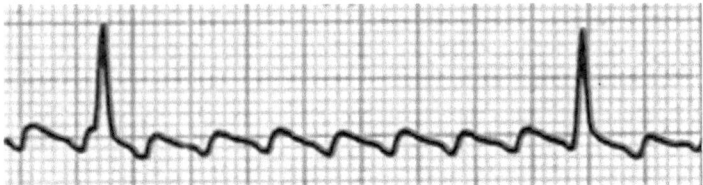

FIGURE 3.8 ECG strip showing atrial flutter with a high ratio of atrial to ventricular conduction resulting in a saw tooth appearance

rhythm that occurs with atrial rates exceeding 300 bpm, the atrial rate in atrial flutter is slower due to a larger circuit. This has important implications as each flutter wave has the potential under certain conditions to conduct through the AV node in a 1:1 fashion, as dictated by the conductivity of the AV node and atrial rate, that could result in dangerously fast heart rates which may deteriorate into VF. Conductivity through the AV node is increased by sympathetic tone. Therefore, patients in atrial flutter should be guided by a specialist regarding exercise, particularly in athletes. Furthermore, class 1c antiarrhythmic drugs e.g. Flecainide, should be combined with an AV nodal blocker such as a beta-blocker or calcium channel blocker as class 1c agents are known to slow the atrial rate which may then be conducted in a 1:1 fashion, leading paradoxically to higher ventricular rates. In contrast to AF, catheter ablation for common atrial flutter is a shorter, simpler procedure that is well tolerated under local anaesthetic with approximately 95 % success rate with a much lower risk of complications. It is performed via the femoral vein and ablation is performed to break the flutter circuit at a critical point where it runs between the tricuspid annulus and the inferior vena cava – the cavotricuspid isthmus. Unlike AF ablation, many patients can discontinue antiarrhythmic therapy and anticoagulation post ablation providing there is no co-existing AF. Due to the favourable benefit:risk ratio, the threshold for recommending ablation in atrial flutter at an earlier stage is much lower.

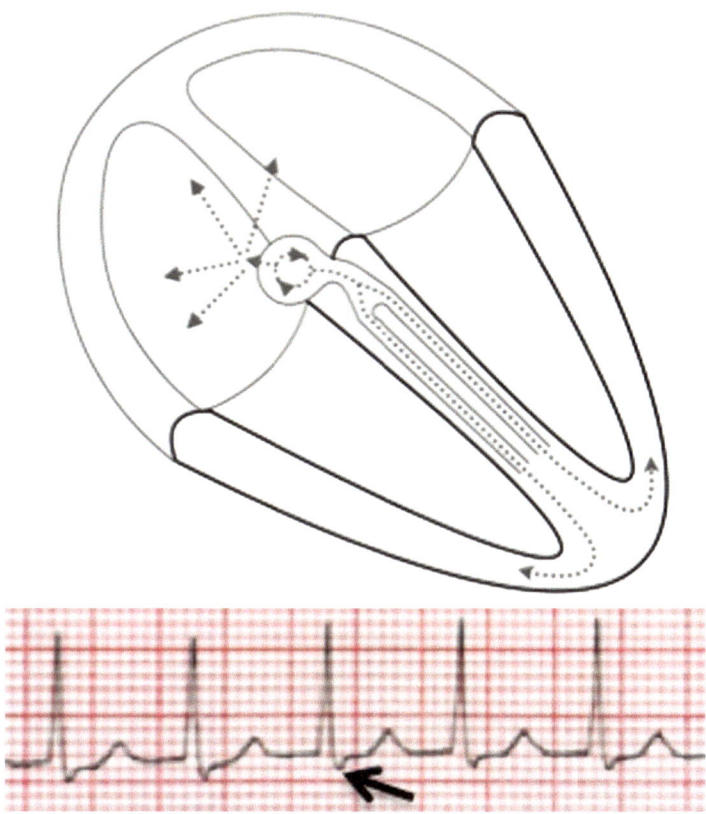

FIGURE 3.9 *Top panel*: Illustration of the mechanism of atrioventricular nodal tachycardia. *Bottom panel*: ECG of atrioventricular nodal tachycardia demonstrating retrograde inverted p waves (*arrow*) at the end of the QRS complex

Supraventricular Tachycardias

Supraventricular tachycardia is a term commonly applied to a group of arrhythmias that encompasses AVNRT (Fig. 3.9), AVRT (also referred to as accessory pathway mediated tachycardia; Fig. 3.10) and AT (Fig. 3.11). They are common arrhythmias that can be recurrent, but are rarely fatal and most often occur in

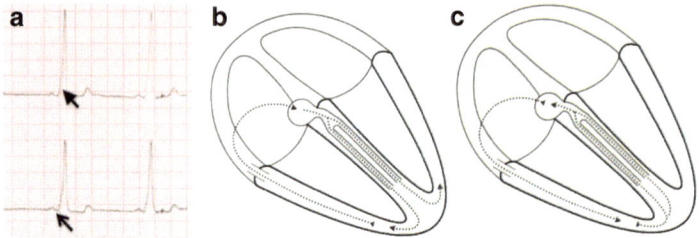

FIGURE 3.10 Panel **a**: Sinus rhythm pre-excited ECG demonstrating a short PR interval (*open arrow head*) and slurred upstroke of the QRS complex – delta wave (*closed arrow head*). Panel **b**: Diagram illustrating the mechanism of orthodromic tachycardia. Panel **c**: Diagram illustrating the mechanism of antidromic tachycardia

the setting of a structurally normal heart. Fifteen percent of SVTs can present as syncope either just after initiation or termination with a prolonged pause. They usually manifest as a narrow complex tachycardia when recorded on ECG. Exceptions to this are when they are conducted aberrantly due to underlying bundle branch block or when conduction occurs from atria to ventricles (antegradely) over an accessory pathway. Of these rhythms, only pre-excitation due to an accessory pathway can reliably be diagnosed on an ECG in sinus rhythm. Capturing an ECG during tachycardia can be problematic but when achieved, can provide clues as to the underlying diagnosis. Further clues can be gained from examining the initiation and termination of the tachycardia but this is rarely documented. In practice, it is often difficult to diagnose the underlying mechanism of SVT on a surface ECG with any certainty as both the antegrade and retrograde conduction properties of the SVT circuit can vary significantly. Nonetheless, patient demographics and clinical pattern, together with ECG changes may allow diagnosis with reasonable accuracy. When considering incidence alone, AVNRT occurs in approximately 65 %, AVRT in 25 % and AT in 10 % of patients presenting with SVT.

In the acute setting, management of a patient presenting in regular narrow complex tachycardia is usually successful with

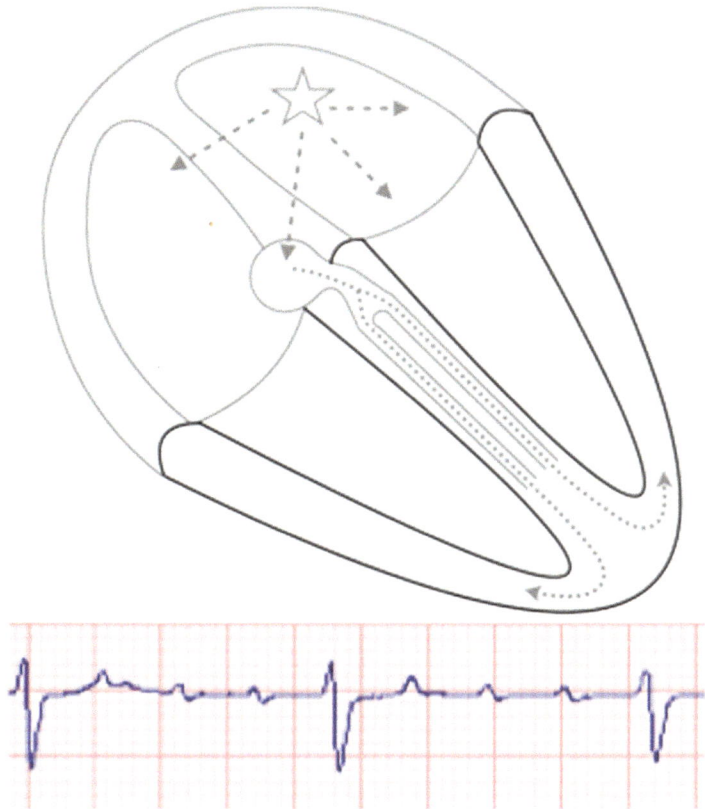

FIGURE 3.11 *Top panel*: Diagram illustrating the mechanism of atrial tachycardia. *Bottom panel*: ECG showing atrial tachycardia with regular P waves separated by isoelectric baseline with a high atrial to ventricular conduction ratio

simple measures. If haemodynamically compromised, then urgent electrical cardioversion should be performed with minimal delay. If stable, then a variety of measures can be undertaken. The AV node is a critical part of the circuit in AVNRT and AVRT, however in AT it is not essential as the atrial focus automatically fires independently. However, the AV node does dictate the ventricular response to an AT. Therapy should therefore be directed at slowing AV nodal conduction regardless of the mechanism. Typically, vagal manoeuvres are tried first and should be done ideally with a continuous 12 lead ECG recording. Secondarily, intravenous AV nodal blocking agents such as adenosine, beta-blockers and calcium channel blockers are effective in the majority of cases in terminating AVRT and AVNRT and may allow better identification of AT as the underlying P waves should be seen on the continuous 12 lead ECG. Adenosine may also terminate AT in 15 % of cases. If further control is needed, intravenous class 1c agents such as Flecaininde or Propafenone can be added. Failing this, electrical cardioversion can be performed, though facilities for emergency cardioversion should be present prior to administration of any pharmacological agent, particularly if there is any suspicion of an accessory pathway being present.

Chronic pharmacological therapy can be used to control symptoms however, for definitive diagnosis and treatment, electrophysiological study (EPS) proceeding to ablation is safe and highly successful in achieving a long-term cure in over 90 % of cases. EPS is typically performed under local anaesthesia using femoral and/or subclavian venous, and occasionally arterial, access to place a number of catheters at critical sites in the atria, ventricles and AV junction to record intracardiac electrical activation. During the study, attempts to induce and study the mechanism of SVT will be made and ablation can proceed thereafter. Studies last on average 2–3 h and are well tolerated by most patients.

Accessory Pathways

Accessory pathways joining atria to ventricle across the AV groove are common. When pre-excitation is seen on the ECG in addition to symptoms from arrhythmia, it constitutes the Wolff-Parkinson-White syndrome (WPW). Accessory pathways can be classified according to their location on the Tricuspid and Mitral annulus and type of conduction. Rarely, multiple pathways in an individual can exist. Conduction

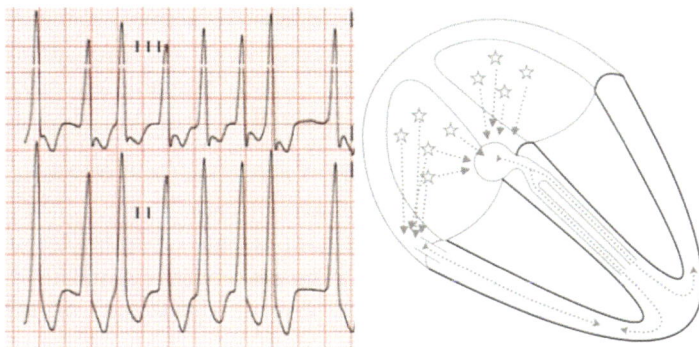

Figure 3.12 *Left panel*: ECG showing pre-excited AF with an irregular broad complex tachycardia in a patient with Wolff-Parkinson-White syndrome. *Right panel*: Diagram illustrating the mechanism of pre-excited AF

properties of accessory pathways can vary with some pathways only capable of anterograde or retrograde conduction or both. Most accessory pathways only conduct in a retrograde direction and so will not be seen on ECG in sinus rhythm (concealed pathway). Furthermore, speed of conduction through the pathway can vary and may slow over time. Depending on the direction that the pathway is able to conduct, it can participate in *orthodromic* tachycardia whereby activation proceeds in the normal (orthodox) direction through the AV node then up the pathway producing a narrow complex on ECG during tachycardia, or *antidromic* tachycardia where activation proceeds first down through the pathway causing a wide complex tachycardia then retrogradely up the AV node to complete the circuit (Fig. 3.10).

Pathways that conduct anterogradely merit particular attention as they have the potential to cause sudden cardiac death in 0.1–0.4 % of patients, which may be the first manifestation of WPW. This is thought to be due to rapid conduction of AF over the pathway, causing unsustainably high rates deteriorating into VF (Fig. 3.12). It is critical in a patient with pre-excited AF that AV node blocking agents are avoided as this may cause the situation to deteriorate due to preferential conduction over the pathway. The risk of sudden death in WPW is related to how rapidly the pathway is able to recover conduction after transmitting an impulse (refractory period). There are a number of tests that may allow the refractory period to be inferred such as exercise testing but can only be determined with any degree of accuracy by performing EPS. American guidelines have recently been updated and recommend that patients with pre-excitation evident on baseline ECG, in whom an exercise test shows that it does not disappear at faster sinus rates, should undergo EPS with a view to curative ablation if the pathway is able to conduct at dangerously fast rates (typically refractory period of 220–250 ms). Importantly, unevaluated/untreated patients with WPW should be advised against exercise.

Ventricular Ectopics

Ventricular ectopics (VEs) are a very common cause of palpitations and reason for referral to specialist clinics. In general, if they are infrequent and not associated with structural heart disease, they carry a benign prognosis and reassurance is all that is required. Occasionally, if VEs are very frequent i.e. when they comprise more than 10–20 % of the total beats in a 24 h period, in a number of patients, this can lead to a form of cardiomyopathy and heart failure if sustained over a long period. These patients require further evaluation as treatment of VEs pharmacologically or by catheter ablation can reverse heart failure in a selected group.

Ventricular Tachycardia

Sustained monomorphic VT is a potentially life-threatening rhythm that most commonly occurs in the context of myocardial scar which can be formed by several disease processes, of which the most common is myocardial infarction. There should

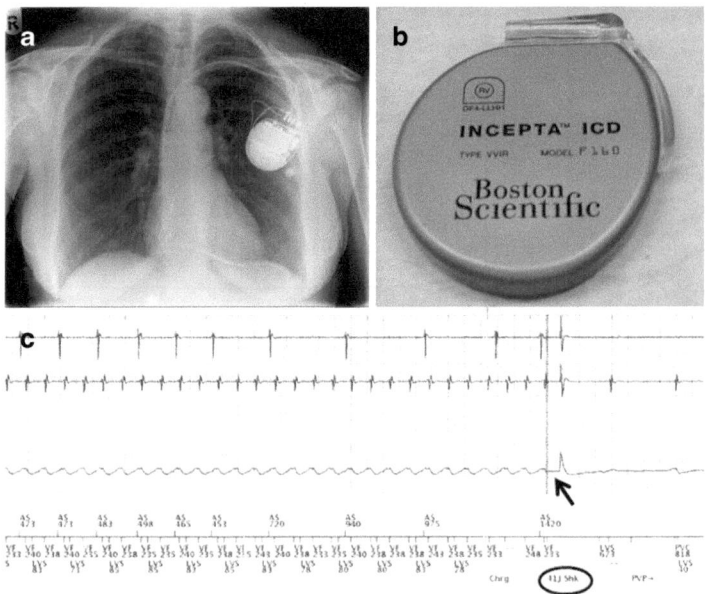

FIGURE 3.13 Panel **a**: Chest X-ray showing an implanted dual chamber single coil ICD with leads in the right atrium and right ventricle. Panel **b**: ICD generator. Panel **c**: Trace recorded by an ICD of a fast ventricular tachycardia treated with a shock (*arrow and circle*)

therefore be a low index of suspicion in patients presenting with palpitations or syncope in these high risk patients. Symptoms can vary widely from mild breathlessness to haemodynamic collapse and cardiac arrest. Patients with implantable cardioverter-defibrillators (ICDs) are a special group identified to be at high risk of recurrent VT and sudden death. Defibrillators work by detecting the onset of VT which triggers therapies through the device such as overdrive pacing or shock therapy to terminate VT (Fig. 3.13). The threshold for triggering therapies from the device is manually programmed. This is important as it is still possible for a patient with a defibrillator in place to have VT despite not having any apparent therapy delivered such as in the case of a slower, more haemodynamically tolerated VT.

TABLE 3.9 ECG features of ventricular tachycardia

Capture and fusion beats
Very wide QRS >160 ms
North-west frontal plane axis
Positive or negative concordance across V1-V6
Absence of a typical RBBBB or LBBB pattern

In patients with suspected VT, correct identification is essential as treatments used for other arrhythmias are potentially harmful. As a general rule, any broad complex tachycardia should be assumed to be VT if in doubt and managed appropriately. An ECG during sinus rhythm is useful and may provide clues to the underlying disease process (Table 3.2). The main differential diagnosis of a broad complex tachycardia is SVT with aberrant conduction or pre-excited tachycardia. Many criteria have been developed to distinguish VT from SVT with aberrancy which in some cases can be challenging even to a specialist; however as a rule of thumb, VT is a much more common cause of broad complex tachycardia. Diagnosis of VT can be made by examining the ECG for subtle signs of ventricular activation occurring independently of atrial activation (AV dissociation) and grossly abnormal activation patterns that indicate that ventricular depolarization does not start or spread in a normal direction (Table 3.9).

In haemodynamically unstable VT, electrical cardioversion is always appropriate. In more stable forms, acute intravenous antiarrhythmic therapy can involve beta-blockade, amiodarone or lidocaine. As VT can be adrenergically driven, one important measure in recurrent VT is rapid sedation and in refractory cases, general anaesthesia may be indicated. This can be useful, particularly in patients who are having frequent shocks from implantable defibrillators in whom repeated shocks cause significant distress which leads to further shocks. Chronic treatment usually involves long-term therapy with amiodarone or mexiletine. Implantation of an ICD may also be appropriate. Despite the success of ICDs in reducing mortality in patients with isch-aemic heart disease, frequent shocks occur despite optimal use of antiarrhythmics which can be debilitating and are associated with significant morbidity and hospitalization. ICDs can only treat VT when it occurs but are not preventa-tive. Catheter ablation of VT in these patients has been shown to reduce the frequency of shocks but require long procedures under general anaesthetic with associated risks.

Conclusion

Palpitations are a common symptom in patients presenting to primary and secondary care. Causes are wide and whilst most carry a benign prognosis, identification of underlying condi-tions that are potentially life threatening is mandatory. Commonly used antiarrhythmics need careful consideration before prescribing in view of their risks of proarrhythmia particularly where there is underlying heart disease. Catheter ablation is being increasingly used in patients with arrhyth-mia affording the potential for cure in many arrhythmias.

Guidelines

European guidelines on the management of AF
    http://www.escardio.org/guidelines-surveys/esc-guidelines/ Pages/atrial-fibrillation.aspx
    European guidelines on the management of SVT
    http://www.escardio.org/guidelines-surveys/esc-guidelines/ Pages/supraventricular-arrhythmias.aspx
    American guidelines on the management of WPW
    http://www.hrsonline.org/Practice-Guidance/ Clinical-Guidelines-Documents/2012-Management-of-the-Asymptomatic-Young-Patient-with-a-Wolff-Parkinson-White#axzz2jOa54qXz

Information for Patients

BHF heart rhythms booklet

http://www.bhf.org.uk/publications/view-publication.aspx?ps=1001001

BHF Atrial fibrillation booklet

http://www.bhf.org.uk/publications/view-publication.aspx?ps=1000952

BHF information on electrophysiological studies

http://www.bhf.org.uk/heart-health/tests/electrophysiology-studies.aspx

Chapter 4
Syncope

Hariharan Raju and Elijah R. Behr

Introduction

Syncope is a common symptom in the general population, reflected by the lifetime prevalence of between 30 and 50 %. Therefore, it is imperative that non-specialists identify and reassure those with relatively benign conditions such as reflex (neurally-mediated) syncope, while referring those at risk of injury and/or sudden death for specialist advice and management. This chapter will focus on reflex and cardiac-related syncope.

Differential Diagnosis

Syncope is part of the spectrum of presentations frequently referred to as "fits, faints and funny turns" (Fig. 4.1) and fits within the differential diagnosis for transient loss of consciousness (T-LOC). Specifically, the term syncope should be reserved for T-LOC that occurs due to global cerebral hypoperfusion. However, in some circumstances, the initial

H. Raju • E.R. Behr, MA, MBBS, MD, FRCP (✉)
Cardiovascular Sciences Research Centre,
Cardiovascular and Cell Sciences Research Institute,
St George's University of London, London SW17 0RE, UK
e-mail: drhraju@doctors.org.uk; ebehr@sgul.ac.uk

J.C. Kaski et al. (eds.), *Investigating and Managing Common Cardiovascular Conditions*, DOI 10.1007/978-1-4471-6696-2_4,
© Springer-Verlag London 2015

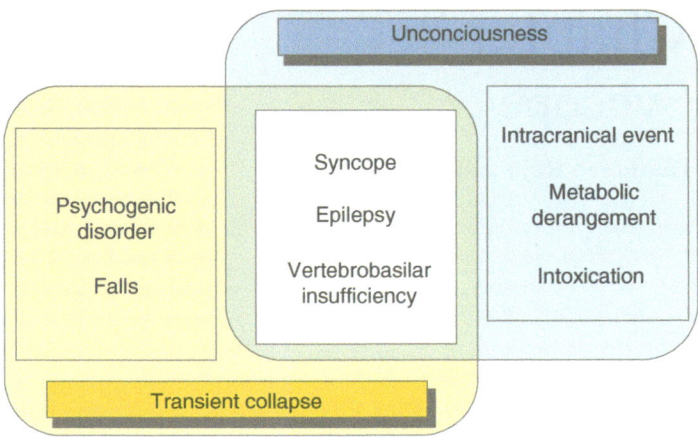

FIGURE 4.1 Presentations that may be categorised as fits, faints (unconsciousness) or funny turns, including collapse query cause (transient collapse). True transient loss of consciousness differential diagnosis is represented in the central white box

presentation may be as broad as "collapse query cause" thereby requiring a more circumspect approach to diagnosis.

True syncope has a number of potential underlying causes, detailed in Fig. 4.2 and divided by mechanism. It is important to have an accurate early clinical impression of any presentation, in order to avoid inappropriate investigation or reassurance of individuals.

Approaching the Patient with Syncope

A summary of evaluation findings and indicators of necessity for specialist evaluation following syncope are given in Fig. 4.3. Each aspect of the initial evaluation is detailed below.

History

Differentiation between causes of T-LOC is predominantly achieved by careful history-taking, with up to 95 % correctly diagnosed on symptoms alone. Patients may use a variety of

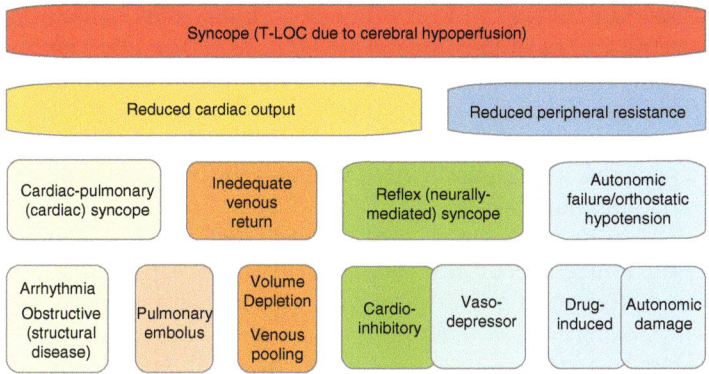

FIGURE 4.2 Potential underlying causes of cardiac syncope, grouped vertically by physiological mechanism for cerebral hypoperfusion

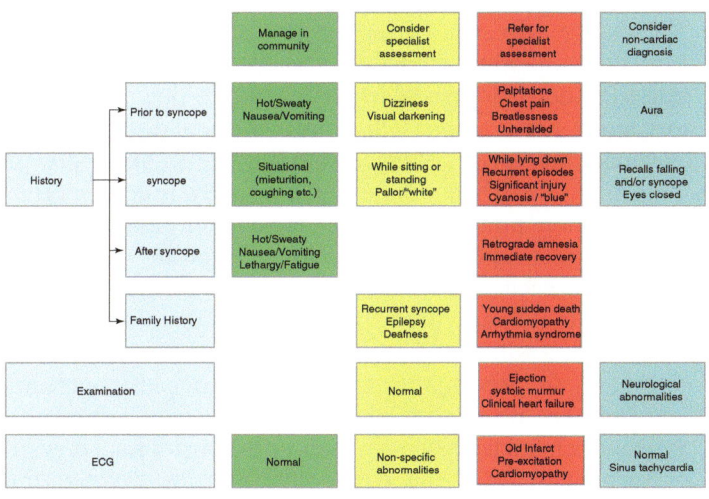

FIGURE 4.3 Suggested clinical indicators of necessity for specialist cardiac referral following presentation with syncope

terms including "blackout" and "faint" to describe an episode of T-LOC. However, the clinician is often hindered by the inability of patients to describe events accurately; witness observations can equally be unreliable or absent in many cases.

Amnesia surrounding the event itself indicates a high likelihood of T-LOC rather than fall, although bear in mind that elderly patients or those with a head injury may be unaware of the extent of unconsciousness due to retrograde amnesia. Hence, individuals initially assessed under the catch-all "collapse query cause" may require careful consideration, since therapeutic interventions aimed at minimising recurrent syncopal risk will be ineffective against falls due to mechanical and ambulatory factors.

Despite the limitations of patient recollection, it is important to ask specifically about events immediately preceding and after any T-LOC. Moreover, you should attempt to elicit a personal and witness description of the period of unconsciousness to facilitate diagnosis. Personal and family medical history can also be useful in risk-stratification.

Circumstances of Syncope

Reflex, or neurally-mediated syncope, the most common cause in adults, is particularly amenable to diagnosis on history alone. For example: fear, pain, emotional distress, clinical instrumentation or prolonged standing are frequent precipitants. Syncope while supine is very rarely reflex in origin, except when precipitated by such an emotional stimulus. Prodromes of reflex syncope include symptoms of increased vagal tone such as nausea, vomiting, sweating and general fatigue. Situational syncope, which shares an autonomic aetiology, occurs with coughing, swallowing, micturition or defecation; these precipitants are thought to cause increased intrathoracic pressure and subsequent vagal stimulation. Syncope related to shaving in men, or during looking upwards or turning to cross the street may indicate carotid sinus hypersensitivity, another form of neurally-mediated syncope.

Syncope during active exercise is rarely reflex in origin, although the typical increase in parasympathetic tone immediately post-exercise can be responsible for syncope. This post-exertional effect can unmask orthostatic hypotension, where individuals with true autonomic failure are unable to mount a blood pressure response to exercise, but do suffer from the physiological drop in recovery after exertion. However, post-exertional hypotension and bradycardia are common and normal findings in trained athletes who, at onset of exertion, demonstrate rapid increases in heart rate and blood pressure, with similar precipitous falls on resting afterward. Orthostatic hypotension is precipitated by standing, though the drop in blood pressure and resultant syncope may be delayed by several minutes after posture change. While autonomic in origin, orthostatic hypotension is due to disease of the autonomic system rather than an inappropriate reflex in health. Therefore, the prodrome of reflex syncope is absent. A rare variant of autonomic failure can present with post-prandial syncope, particularly with high carbohydrate loads. Dehydration and hot environment (due to skin vasodilation) increase risk for orthostatic hypotension, though this may also contribute to reflex syncope.

Arrhythmic and other cardiac syncope may occur with little or no warning, referred to as unheralded. Alternatively, sudden onset palpitations, indicative of paroxysmal tachyarrhythmia may precede the event. Syncope during exercise or exertion, but excluding early post-exercise syncope, is highly suggestive of a primary cardiac cause.

Epilepsy, an important differential for T-LOC, may be preceded by a stereotypical aura, often specific to the individual. These may include a rising epigastric sensation, distinctive smell or taste, deja vu, or visual aura (but not generally visual field loss or blurring, which are more likely to indicate cardiovascular syncope). Epilepsy may be precipitated by flashing lights, such as during video-game playing and is also seen during sleep deprivation.

Period of Loss of Consciousness

During the period of unconsciousness, the patient should have no recollection of events. If he or she can recall events from the period of unresponsiveness, psychogenic (or non-epileptic) attacks are the most likely diagnosis.

Unresponsiveness lasting a long time (more than 2 or 3 min) also suggests a psychogenic cause; this is often associated with waxing and waning of prominent limb and pelvic thrusting. Another useful indicator of psychogenic cause is that the patient's eyes are generally closed during the episode, unlike syncope and epilepsy, where the eyes remain open. Moreover, about 10 % of psychogenic blackouts initially present with mimicry of status epilepticus.

Epileptic attacks vary in appearance, however, depending on the type of seizure. Generalised seizures are often seen as initial rigidity and fixed extension of limbs, with subsequent symmetrical tonic-clonic limb movements of large amplitude, which gradually decrease in amplitude over the course of the seizure. Importantly, limb movements may commence prior to loss of consciousness, which is not seen in syncope. They very rarely last longer than 1 min, although panicked bystanders may overestimate the duration when reporting collateral history. Biting of the lateral tongue border (rather than tip) and frothing mouth are other signs of generalised epilepsy. Facial cyanosis may also be seen, although cyanosis can equally indicate malignant arrhythmia. Complex partial seizures may present with asymmetric or unilateral twitching, head-turning or lip-smacking; altered consciousness may be present at onset, or become apparent later during the attack. Secondary generalisation, with features akin to generalised epilepsy, may be witnessed.

Limb jerking and other mimics of seizures can occur with syncope, due to secondary cerebral hypoxia. It is important to appreciate this so as to avoid the pitfall of diagnosing a primary seizure in these cases. In fact, they are associated with convulsive syncope of any aetiology, including reflex syncope. Extreme facial pallor, described by witnesses as, "white as a sheet," while frightening to bystanders, is also indicative of the central vasodilation and preferential vascular flow away from the skin of reflex syncope. In contrast, individuals who experience arrhythmic syncope may be cyanotic, though this appearance is also seen in epileptic seizures. Syncopal loss of consciousness is less than 30 s in duration and generally less than 15 s.

Return of Consciousness

Post-event recovery following epileptic seizures can take over 5 min, with prolonged confusion and disorientation; other features include headache and muscle ache, though bruising due to a fall may confound this symptom. Recovery from reflex syncope is more rapid, although similar autonomic post-event symptoms to the prodrome are frequent, particularly prolonged fatigue and lethargy. In the absence of physical injury, resumption of normal activity following arrhythmic syncope is generally instantaneous, such that patients may not recognise the seriousness of the event. Other cardiac causes of syncope may leave individuals with associated residual symptoms such as breathlessness, chest pain or palpitations.

Past Medical and Medication History

Syncope that occurs in the context of structural or functional heart disease is most likely to be secondary to malignant arrhythmia. Loss of consciousness in individuals with alcoholism, autism, cerebral palsy, learning difficulties or brain injury tends to associate with epilepsy. Primary nervous system disease such as multisystem atrophy and systemic diseases with neuropathic complications, such as diabetic and amyloid neuropathy suggest orthostatic hypotension; this may be exacerbated by medications such as antihypertensives, antidepressants and diuretics. However, antidepressants may also result in cardiac depolarisation and repolarisation anomalies which predispose to malignant arrhythmias, so this should always be considered. Other medications, alcohol and drugs of abuse are also know to affect cardiac electrophysiology adversely, especially in overdose.

Family History

Family history may provide an important marker for more malignant syncope. Close blood relatives of individuals with inherited primary arrhythmia syndromes (e.g. long QT syndrome, Brugada syndrome and catecholaminergic polymorphic tachycardia) or inherited myocardial disorders (e.g. hypertrophic cardiomyopathy, familial dilated cardiomyopathy, arrhythmogenic right ventricular cardiomyopathy) who present with transient loss of consciousness should be thoroughly investigated for these conditions, since the risk of sudden death is high. Similarly, a family history of premature and/or unexplained sudden death may represent undiagnosed cardiovascular genetic conditions in up to half of all cases and should prompt comprehensive cardiac evaluation for inherited disease. A family history of recurrent seizures or epilepsy warrants close evaluation for both familial epilepsy and inherited cardiac conditions, due to the possibility of misdiagnosis of syncope as epilepsy.

Examination

Clinical examination can suggest specific cardiac or neurological causes for syncope, though the vast majority of patients have normal findings especially in reflex syncope.

Obstruction to left ventricular outflow, caused either by hypertrophic cardiomyopathy or aortic stenosis, may be diagnosed clinically by the character of an ejection systolic murmur, in addition to the changes with squatting and/or amplitude of the second heart sound. Similarly atrial myxoma may be suggested by a tumour plop or mitral valve murmur. Signs of heart failure are less specific, though do indicate a likely cardiac cause. Significant difference in bilateral arm blood pressures may suggest aortic pathology, though it may indicate a possible subclavian steal in syncopal patients.

Any focal neurological deficits are strongly suggestive of epilepsy. However, limb weakness, ataxia and cranial nerve dysfunction may indicate vertebrobasilar transient ischaemic attacks (TIA). In general, TIA should not be considered in the differential for syncope in the absence of a coinciding suggestive neurological deficit.

Postural blood pressures should be measured in any individuals where orthostatic hypotension is suspected. Orthostatic hypotension is defined as a 20 mmHg drop in systolic or 10 mmHg drop in diastolic blood pressure within 3 min of standing. It is therefore readily identified by bedside clinical examination. Some individuals suffer a delayed fall in blood pressure and repeat recording 3 min after standing may be necessary.

ECG

A 12-lead ECG is mandatory in all syncopal individuals. The diagnostic yield is low, since reflex syncope, the most common cause, is usually associated with a normal ECG. However, this is an important negative finding, necessary for appropriate reassurance.

Pathological changes on the ECG are highly suggestive of a cardiac cause of syncope (commonly ventricular tachyarrhythmias or bradycardia) and an abnormal ECG is an independent predictor of subsequent mortality but is treatable in a majority. Signs of myocardial, primary arrhythmic, valvular and cardiac conduction system disease may be present on the resting ECG as well as prior myocardial infarction.

ECG examples of rare but life-threatening primary arrhythmia syndromes are provided. Figure 4.4 illustrates the typical type 1 Brugada ECG pattern, with coved ST elevation and T wave inversion in the right ventricular leads, which may be mistaken for acute myocardial infarction. Figure 4.5 illustrates a patient with long QT syndrome, which may be induced or exacerbated by medication that prolongs the QT interval. Wolff-Parkinson-White (see Chapter 3) can also be potentially fatal if associated with a paroxysm of pre-excited atrial fibrillation involving a rapidly conducting accessory pathway. This may have reverted to sinus by the time of ECG recording. Hypertrophic cardiomyopathy is suggested by ST depression associated with deep T wave inversion in the lateral ECG leads (Fig. 4.6).

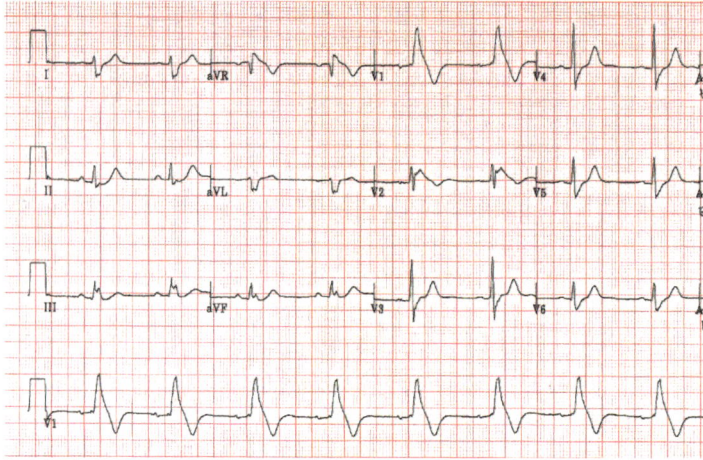

FIGURE 4.4 12-lead ECG of a patient with Brugada syndrome demonstrating type 1 pattern in V1 and V2. Inferior early repolarisation is also present

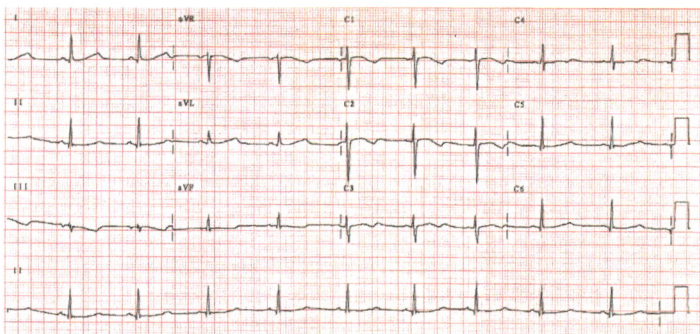

FIGURE 4.5 12-lead ECG of a patient with congenital long QT syndrome (type 2) demonstrating inverted and/or notched T waves in precordial leads associated with QT prolongation

Other Investigations

Additional investigations are focussed on identification of arrhythmic and epileptic features. Ambulatory ECG monitoring provides the possibility for correlation of symptoms

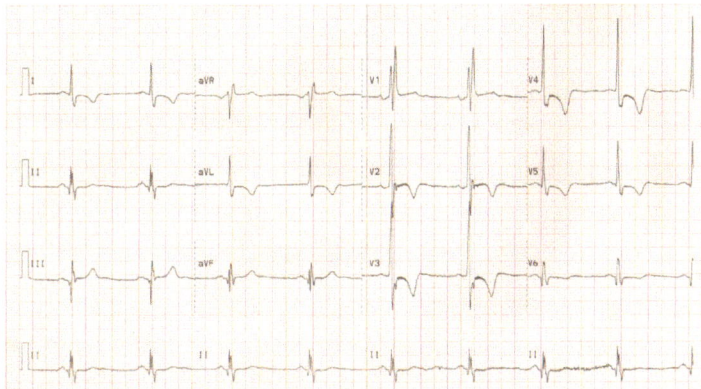

FIGURE 4.6 12-lead ECG of a patient with hypertrophic cardiomy-opathy showing ST depression and deep T wave inversion in affected myocardial territories (septal). Right bundle branch block is also present

with arrhythmia. Historically, 24-h monitoring has been used for this purpose. However, it has a diagnostic yield of only around 1 %, due to the relatively short duration of monitoring, and the low likelihood of documenting a syncopal episode. Moreover, the possibility for erroneous reassurance, or inappropriate attribution of syncope to asymptomatic arrhythmias, can make this an unhelpful addition. Holter monitoring for several days only improves this yield marginally, while patients struggle to document cardiac rhythm with handheld event recorders during symptoms. Outside the context of arrhythmic syncope, ambulatory monitoring is unnecessary.

In those where arrhythmic syncope is suspected but undocumented the implantable loop recorder provides the opportunity for safe delay of therapy until documentation; a similar strategy can also be successful in the diagnosis of reflex syncope with an atypical history. The implantable loop recorder is placed under local anaesthesia in the prepectoral fascia of the left chest wall. It measures approximately 6 cm × 2 cm × 1 cm, and is generally unobtrusive in this position. Unlike a pacemaker, it requires no intravascular or intracardiac connections, reducing potential for device complication. The battery contained within it lasts 18–24 months, and it is able to document heart rhythm during syncope in about 90 % of individuals.

Tilt-Table Testing

Tilt-table testing can produce typical reflex syncope and thereby confirm prior suspicion especially in cases where there is coexistent and potentially life-threatening cardiac disease. However, a tilt response is not necessarily reproducible when repeated in the same patient and can be induced in an asymptomatic person. Moreover, the specific response seen (e.g. bradycardia of cardio-inhibitory type or hypotension of vasodepressor type) may not reflect the predominant mechanism in spontaneous syncope. Therefore, tailoring of treatment cannot be reliably performed. Tilt-testing does allow the opportunity for parallel recording of haemodynamics, ECG and EEG. This can prove useful in suggestible patients affected by psychogenic syncope, where documentation of normal physiology during attacks can confirm the diagnosis.

Cardiac Imaging

Echocardiography, cardiac CT and cardiac magnetic resonance (CMR) imaging have differing but complementary strengths in cardiac imaging. The relative merits of each modality are beyond the scope of this chapter. However, as with ECG recordings, cardiac structure and function is normal in most cases of T-LOC. While the combination of a normal ECG and echocardiogram arguably strengthens the evidence for favourable prognosis, the incremental benefit in the context of a normal ECG is minimal. Therefore, except where the history is suggestive of arrhythmic syncope, or where the ECG is abnormal, cardiac imaging is of uncertain benefit.

Neurological Investigation

As with syncope, epilepsy is in most circumstances a clinical diagnosis, made with personal and collateral history alongside physical examination findings. Brain imaging (with CT or MRI) and EEG can strengthen the diagnosis, though their main role is differentiation between different forms of epilepsy and prognostic indication of recurrent seizures. It is of specific importance in those with a history of focal (partial) seizures or focal neurological deficits on examination. The EEG has recognised limitations, and sleep-deprived EEG or video EEG may improve both sensitivity and specificity. Overall, brain imaging is generally an overused investigation in those presenting acutely with T-LOC.

Role for Specialist Referrals

Most presentations with syncope can safely be managed as an outpatient and admission from the Emergency Department are generally unwarranted. Prognosis is favourable for reflex syncope. Therefore, these individuals can be reassured and discharged although outpatient assessment by a cardiologist or syncope specialist may be necessary (Fig. 4.3). Early discharge of patients with syncope is not advised in the following situations: recurrent frequent syncope; syncope during exertion; syncope during palpitations; significant personal injury; personal history of cardiac disease; family history of premature sudden unexpected death or inherited heart disease; ECG anomalies indicating structural or arrhythmic risk. Specific indicators of risk include: prior myocardial infarction or heart failure; advanced conduction system disease; primary arrhythmia syndromes; pre-excitation and/or Wolff-Parkinson-White syndrome. These risk factors are identifiable by history and ECG; inpatient evaluation by a cardiologist is warranted in these situations.

Importantly, unless a clinical diagnosis of seizure is made, brain imaging is unnecessary. Where a diagnosis of epilepsy is suspected, the indication for urgent inpatient brain imaging is dependent on the likelihood of acute neurological illness or injury; the diagnosis of epilepsy is beyond the scope of this book. Suspicion of epilepsy should prompt referral to a neurologist to confirm the diagnosis.

Diagnostic Challenges

Occasionally, serious acute cardiovascular conditions can present with syncope as the predominant symptom. This includes acute myocardial infarction or pulmonary embolism. Specifically, haemodynamic compromise causing syncope can result from ischaemic arrhythmia or sudden increase in right ventricular afterload respectively. The presence of chest pain or breathlessness either preceeding or after syncope should be taken seriously and prompt careful evaluation for these disorders. Firstly, both conditions are likely to associate with ECG anomalies. Repolarisation anomalies such as ST or T wave changes should raise myocardial ischaemia as a potential cause. Pulmonary embolism is classically described as causing an "SI, QIII, TIII" pattern. i.e. deep S in lead I, deep Q and T inversion in lead III; however, this is a rare finding, and sinus tachycardia, right bundle branch block or delay and T wave changes in right precordial leads (V1 to V3) are more commonly seen. Additional investigations that may assist in making these diagnoses include biomarkers (e.g. troponin and D-dimers), chest radiograph, arterial pO_2 and echocardiography.

FAQ

My patient with classical reflex syncope has suffered significant facial injury. What should I do?

Significant injury is unusual in reflex syncope, but can occur. In this case, specialist referral is warranted to confirm the diagnosis and offer medical and/or device therapy as appropriate.

I've documented a significant sinus pause on ambulatory monitoring. Does my patient need a pacemaker?

Maybe. Correlation of symptomatic presyncope or syncope with sinus pauses is generally considered an indication for permanent pacemaker implantation. Nocturnal and asymptomatic pauses are not an immediate indication. If the pauses are neurally-mediated, they often coincide with neurally-mediated vasodilation and therefore hypotension, which aggravates symptoms. Pacing may alleviate the bradycardia but not the hypotension in these episodes, which often means less frequent and less severe symptoms, but not necessarily complete abolition of symptoms. Particular care needs to be taken in recommending pacemakers for reflex syncope in those aged below 40 years, due to the potential for late device complications throughout life.

Are there special pacemakers for reflex syncope?

Yes, but they are still not 100 % effective at preventing symptoms. So-called rate-drop algorithms in some dual-chamber pacemakers will compensate for sudden neurally-mediated bradycardic (cardio-inhibitory) episodes by pacing at approximately 100 beats per minute, which increases cardiac output sufficiently to compensate for the coincident vasodilation. However, some individuals suffer such bradycardic episodes at night, and initiation of pacing at such high rates can cause symptomatic palpitations.

Which types of heart block require a pacemaker?

Any symptomatic atrioventricular heart block should be considered for pacemaker therapy, particularly if there are no contributary medications and neurally-mediated syncope is considered unlikely. Correlation of symptoms with bradycardia is important in decision-making if demonstrable, though this is often not possible. Evidence of conduction disease, including combinations of first degree block, left or right bundle branch block, in the context of probable arrhythmic syncope, may be considered sufficient evidence for recommendation of pacemaker, particularly in older individuals. Asymptomatic high degree atrioventricular block such as second degree Mobitz type II and complete (third degree) heart block generally require pacemaker implantation, irrespective of medication taken, and should be referred urgently for cardiological evaluation.

Aren't highly-trained athletes prone to bradycardia and associated syncope?

Yes. Athletes have a high resting vagal tone, predisposing them to neurally-mediated syncope, often immediately post-exertion. They may also demonstrate varying degrees of sinus bradycardia and atrioventricular block at rest (including apparent high degree block), which improves with exercise. Such individuals should be assessed by a specialist in sports cardiology in order to determine if therapy is required, or if their response represents physiological cardiac adaptation to exercise.

My patient with syncope had a myocardial infarction years ago, evidenced by Q waves on ECG, but there is no evidence of a recent ischaemic event. Do I need to worry?

Yes. Prior infarctions leave myocardial scarring, which act as the substrate for reentry arrhythmias such as ventricular tachycardia. Such individuals require imaging of ventricular size and systolic function and urgent specialist assessment for consideration of implantable cardioverter defibrillator (ICD). Cardiomyopathies, including dilated, hypertrophic and arrhythmogenic cardiomyopathies, similarly cause scarring and predispose to life-threatening ventricular arrhythmias.

My patient has previously been asymptomatic with pre-excitation (delta wave) on ECG, but has now had a syncopal episode. What should I do?

These individuals should be assessed emergently by a specialist in case their syncope represents pre-excited atrial fibrillation that was self-limiting and spontaneously resolved by the time of ECG acquisition.

My patient with syncope has a prolonged QT interval and/or unusual ST/T changes. I wonder if it represents a primary arrhythmia syndrome or possibly a cardiomyopathy. What should I do?

Repolarisation abnormalities on the resting ECG can be indicative of either myocardial disease or primary arrhythmia syndrome. The first priority is to identify arrhythmic precipitants such as electrolyte imbalance, proarrhythmic drugs and other environmental factors such as pyrexia in Brugada syndrome. Drugs implicated in arrhythmia may be illicit (such as cocaine or amphetamines), social (such as alcohol) or prescribed (many potential culprits including antidysrhythmics, antipsychotics, antidepressants and others as listed on websites qtdrugs.org and brugadadrugs.org). With the exception of Brugada syndrome, beta-blockade is indicated in all conditions. However, specialist assessment for consideration of ICD and formal risk assessment as an inpatient is appropriate following syncope.

My patient with syncope has a prolonged QT interval but has an absolute indication for his antipsychotic medication that I think is responsible. What should I do?

This is a difficult clinical conundrum. A balanced decision between psychiatric and cardiac specialists taking into account their arrhythmic risk and options for alternative antipsychotic medications is imperative. If the corrected QT remains below 500 ms and absolute QT less than 600 ms, addition of a beta-blocker to shorten QT interval with continued monitoring *may* be appropriate.

My patient with syncope has a murmur. What should I do?

A clinical murmur should be evaluated in case it represents cardiac pathology. Possible associations include severe aortic stenosis or hypertrophic cardiomyopathy, which can cause syncope due to outflow tract obstruction and reduction in cardiac output or myocardial ischaemia. Mitral valve prolapse can occasionally be associated with ventricular arrhythmias, although this is rare.

What do I tell the patient with reflex syncope?

Describing the diagnosis

Reflex syncope is known by a number of different names, with subgroup definitions that are sometimes used interchangeably; these include vasovagal, neurocardiogenic and neurally-mediated syncope as well as carotid sinus hypersensitivity. These terms describe the unexpected interaction between brain, nerves, heart and blood vessels that cause reflex syncope. In essence, an inappropriate signal is sent to lower your blood pressure and heart rate, but your brain and nervous system are otherwise completely normal.

Appropriate reassurance

Reflex syncope is the most common cause of T-LOC and affects up to half of all people at some point in their life. It is readily managed by simple measures and only a small minority of those affected require ongoing active medical therapy. Although approximately one in three affected will go on to have a repeat episode in the 3 years after their initial review, reflex syncope does not portend life-threatening events.

Therapeutic Options

Many people require no regular therapy. For example, those with infrequent episodes should be advised to lie down during the prodrome and leave any warm indoor environment safely, if possible. Moreover, active exercise involving lower or upper limbs at this time can abate syncope. Effective mechanisms for this include raising legs with a cycling movement, squatting on heels, and dynamic self-resistance exercise by leg crossing or arm-tensing. Adequate hydration and salt intake reduces frequency of events, as does avoidance of prolonged standing and identified precipitants in situational syncope. Referral to a syncope specialist is appropriate for individuals who suffer significant injury related to reflex syncope, or in those who have no discernible prodrome or warning. This latter presentation is sometimes called the atypical form, which can be difficult to differentiate from other causes of syncope. Pharmacological therapies have universally failed to demonstrate consistent benefits, though midodrine is perhaps the best available option at present. Its use mandates specialist guidance and blood pressure monitoring and it is not licensed in many countries. Other medications which have previously been used, but lack supporting evidence include serotonin reuptake inhibitors (e.g. fluoxetine), fludrocortisone and beta-blockers. Tilt-training, a form of rehabilitation program for reflex syncope can be considered, though this requires significant commitment and motivation from the patient in order to achieve benefits. In severely symptomatic patients with demonstrable symptomatic bradycardia on holter monitoring, carotid sinus massage or on tilt-table provocation, pacemaker implantation with specialist programming may reduce severity of symptoms.

Follow-up and Monitoring

The unpredictability of recurrence of reflex syncope makes routine follow-up of those affected unnecessary. Moreover, additional interventions are unavailable. The best approach is to provide a patient information leaflet detailing appropriate lifestyle measures to encourage adherence and thereby reduce associated morbidity.

Driving

In the UK, the DVLA (Driver and Vehicle Licensing Agency) have rigid guidelines for continued driving following T-LOC. As of 2013, reflex syncope generally requires no restriction to driving cars, though unexplained syncope requires cessation of driving for 6 months. Restrictions for holders of a "Group 2" license are much stricter. Overall, the greater the likelihood of recurrence of loss of consciousness during driving, without warning, the longer the period of license withdrawal.

Red Flags

Syncope in association with the following features deserves emergency inpatient assessment:

  Pre-excitation suggestive of WPW on ECG
  Known history of primary arrhythmia syndrome or cardiomyopathy
  Witnessed cyanosis during episode
  Significant Breathlessness or Chest Pain
  Other associated features warranting specialist assessment include:
  Palpitations
  Unheralded event and immediate recovery
  Audible ejection systolic murmur
  Prior MI or systolic impairment

Also Worth Knowing

Non-ischaemic cardiomyopathies and primary arrhythmias can be associated with ECG anomalies indicative of acute coronary syndromes, and may also cause biomarker elevation in the context of tachyarrhythmia. Such cases should be referred emergently for specialist evaluation to exclude acute myocardial ischaemia in the first instance, and subsequent detailed evaluation for non-ischaemic disorders. Arrhythmogenic right ventricular cardiomyopathy is suggested by T wave inversion in V1 to V3, though a similar right ventricular strain pattern may be seen following pulmonary embolism.

Further Reading

Joint 2009 Consensus of European Society of Cardiology and Heart Rhythm Society on Syncope

Moya A, Sutton R, Ammirati F, et al. Guidelines for the diagnosis and management of syncope (version 2009). Eur Heart J. 2009;30:2631–71.

Patient and Medical Information on Reflex Syncope

Syncope Trust and Reflex Anoxic Seizures (STARS) charitable organisation. Website www.stars.org.uk

UK DVLA guidance on suitability to continue driving. Website www.gov.uk/government/publications/at-a-glance

Chapter 5
Systemic Hypertension

Jennifer Roe and Teck K. Khong

Introduction

Hypertension is recognised as the leading cause of death globally. Worldwide, it has been estimated to affect one billion people and contribute to 9.4 million deaths from cardiovascular disease annually. Health Survey for England estimated that approximately 30 % of adults have hypertension, and that 30 % of these were previously unrecognised and are untreated. Importantly, blood pressure (BP) is a continuously distributed variable and a powerful determinant of long-term mortality. Complications and mortality directly correlate with levels of blood pressure, down to a systolic BP of 115 mmHg.

J. Roe, MBBS
Blood Pressure Unit, St George's Hospital NHS Trust, London, UK
e-mail: jenroe85@gmail.com

T.K. Khong, FRCP, MD, MBA (✉)
Blood Pressure Unit, St George's Hospital NHS Trust, London, UK

Institute of Medical & Biomedical Education,
St George's University of London, London, UK
e-mail: tkhong@sgul.ac.uk

J.C. Kaski et al. (eds.), *Investigating and Managing Common*   125
Cardiovascular Conditions, DOI 10.1007/978-1-4471-6696-2_5,
© Springer-Verlag London 2015

Definition and Classification

Systemic hypertension can be defined as a chronic elevation in arterial blood pressure. NICE defines systemic hypertension as a clinic blood pressure (BP) ≥140/90 mmHg. It can be further classified depending on severity as shown on Table 5.1. If ambulatory or home blood pressure measurements are utilised then lower BP values are accepted: stage 1 hypertension would be consistent with systolic values of 135–149 mmHg and diastolic of 85–94 mmHg; stage 2 hypertension would be consistent with ≥150 mmHg systolic and ≥95 mmHg diastolic.

Measuring BP

Conventional BP Measurements

Blood pressure can be measured indirectly with a manual (mercury or anaeroid) or automated sphygmomanometer. Errors in measurement can arise from technique and also use of un-validated or poorly maintained equipment. It is

TABLE 5.1 Classification of hypertension based on clinic and ambulatory or home BP measurements

	Clinic BP measurement	
Category	Systolic	Diastolic
Optimal	<120	<80
Normal	120–129	80–84
High-normal	130–139	85–89
Stage 1 hypertension	140–159	90–99
Stage 2 hypertension	160–179	100–109
Severe hypertension	≥180	≥110
Accelerated hypertension	≥210	≥130
Malignant hypertension	As above with papilloedema	

important to ensure the correct cuff size is used, and that the inflatable bladder covers at least 80 % of the arm circumference. If the cuff is too small it may underestimate BP.

It is recommended that BP measurement should be performed in a standardised environment to allow for inherent variation in BP. Systolic BP can be altered by up to 20 mmHg by factors such as time of day, posture, emotion, exercise, meals, drugs and temperature. Ensure that the patient is relaxed, seated and rested in a temperate setting and has the arm outstretched and supported in midline of sternum. The correct sized cuff should be applied (arm circumference should be noted on the outside of the cuff) and BP measured with a manual or automated device. It is recommended that patients with atrial fibrillation (AF) have their BP measured manually as current automatic devices are inaccurate when the pulse is irregular.

NICE has issued guidance on optimally obtaining a manual blood pressure reading. The environment should be standardised as above with the correct cuff size applied. Then:

- Palpate the brachial pulse in antecubital fossa
- Rapidly inflate the cuff to 20 mmHg above where the brachial pulse disappears
- Deflate the cuff and note where the pulse reappears. This is an approximation of the systolic pressure
- Re-inflate the cuff until 20 mmHg above where the brachial pulse disappears
- Place the stethoscope over the brachial artery ensuring complete skin contact
- Deflate the cuff at 2–3 mmHg per second listening for Korotokoff sounds. Phase 1 indicates systolic BP and phase 5 diastolic. In some patients (pregnant, children, anaemic and elderly patients) phase 5 is present until 0 mmHg, so phase 4 sounds should be used.

Korotokoff Sounds

   Phase 1: First appearance of faint tapping sounds increasing in intensity lasting for at least 2 consecutive beats.

Phase 2: Auscultatory Gap – sounds soften, swish or disappear for a brief period
Phase 3: Return of sharper sounds
Phase 4: Abrupt muffling of sounds that become soft and blowing in quality
Phase 5: All sounds disappear completely

Ambulatory BP Monitoring (ABPM) and Home BP Monitoring (HBPM)

It is now recommended that patients with possible hypertension based on clinic measurements, borderline readings, or white coat hypertension should be offered ambulatory BP monitoring (ABPM) or home BP monitoring (HBMP). ABPM measures the BP twice per hour during the usual waking hours of the patient. A minimum of 14 readings are needed to make a diagnosis of hypertension. HBPM requires the patient to make 2 BP readings per day while seated, with 2 consecutive readings taken 1 min apart. The HBPM should continue for a minimum of 4 days, ideally 7 before a diagnosis of hypertension is made. Averages of these readings can be used to determine need for medical therapy according to ABPM/HBPM thresholds (see Table 5.1).

Target Organ Damage and Cardiovascular Risk

Assessing target organ damage will aid further cardiovascular risk calculation. For instance, LVH and microalbuminuria are independent risk factors of adverse outcome in patients with hypertension and their presence may prompt more aggressive treatment. Conversely, the presence of acute complications may help define the presence of acute, urgent or malignant hypertension, for which immediate treatment is warranted (Table 5.2).

TABLE 5.2 Acute and chronic target organ damage

Organ	Chronic complications	Acute complications
Cardiac	LVH on ECG/echo, CAD from history or ECG, CCF	MI, pulmonary oedema
Cerebrovascular	TIA, stroke	Intracerebral bleeding, TIA, stroke, posterior reversible encephalopathy syndrome (PRES) (seizure, confusion, coma)
Renal	Microalbuminuria, proteinuria, CKD	Haematuria
Retinal	Hypertensive retinopathy grade 1–4	Papilloedema, haemorrhages
Large vessels	Accelerated atherosclerosis, peripheral vascular disease, aneurysms dilatation	Aortic dissection

Aetiology

Over 90 % of patients with hypertension have essential or primary hypertension. The remainder have an underlying cause such as renal disease, endocrine disease, obstructive sleep apnoea, co-arctation of the aorta or genetic diseases of the adrenal-renal axis causing salt retention. In such cases, hypertension may improve when the underlying disease process is corrected.

Essential Hypertension

Studies estimate that up to 90–95 % of hypertension cases are idiopathic. Physiologically, blood pressure is proportional to cardiac output and peripheral resistance. As such, it is hypothesised that the cause of essential hypertension is a complex interaction of genetic polymorphisms controlling blood volume and vascular resistance with environment and patient's lifestyle (such as raised BMI, smoking status, salt intake and levels of physical activity) combining to cause hypertension.

Secondary Hypertension

Secondary causes of hypertension are rare, but patients may present at a younger age with a more accelerated disease process with or without signs and symptoms of an underlying disease.

Renal disease is the most common cause of secondary hypertension. This includes renal parenchymal disease, glomerulonephritis, chronic pyelonephritis or polycystic kidneys and renovascular disease (renal artery stenosis or fibromuscular dysplasia).

Endocrine disease affecting the adrenal glands is a relatively common cause of secondary hypertension. Aldosterone is a mineralocorticoid and excess will cause active reabsorption of sodium (with passive reabsorption of water) causing blood volume expansion. Causes of mineralocorticoid excess include Conn's syndrome (adrenal ademona), bilateral/congenital adrenal hyperplasia, renin-secreting tumours and glucocorticoid-remediable aldosteronism and may also contribute to hypertension in patients with renal artery stenosis. Corticosteroid excess as seen in Cushing's syndrome and with patients prescribed steroid therapy causes hypertension in a variety of ways, including activation of the renin-angiotensin system, upregulation of vasoactive substances and intrinsic mineralocorticoid activity. Phaeochromocytomas can cause hypertension by episodic excretion of catecholamines, adrenaline and noradrenaline, increasing cardiac output and peripheral resistance. Other endocrine causes include acromegaly, hypo and hyperthyroidism.

Alterations in Aldosterone Metabolism

• Glucocorticoid-remediable aldosteronism: This is an auto-somal dominant gain of function mutation resulting from unequal cross-over and fusion of the regulatory gene for 11-hydroxylase (which is normally under physiological control by ACTH) to the coding region of aldosterone synthase. As a consequence, aldosterone synthase is sensitive to ACTH and suppressed by treatment with exogenous glucocorticoids.
• Congenital adrenal hyperplasia: Thisa is an autosomal recessive disorder of 11β-hydroxylase or 17α-hydroxylase deficiency causing an excess of mineralocorticoids (and deficiency of glucocorticoids)
• Apparent mineralocorticoid excess (AME): autosomal recessive disorder causing inactivation of 11β-hydroxysteroid dehydrogenase type 2. This enzyme usually deactivates cortisol present in the renal tissue to minimise the effect of cortisol on mineralocorticoid receptors. Thus, with the mutation, impaired inactivation of cortisol leads to cortisol receptor intoxication and AME.

Increased Sodium Reabsorption

• Liddle's syndrome: autosomal dominant gain of function mutation in an epithelial sodium channel (ENaC) in the collecting duct, causing excess sodium retention.
• Gordon's Syndrome: autosomal dominant gain of function mutation of WNK1 or WNK4. This inactivates the negative regulators of the thiazide-sensitive sodium chloride co-transporter (NCCT) resulting in a sodium excess within the kidney.

Hypertension is important to recognise in pregnancy and is usually classified as >140/90 or an increase of >30 % from SBP at booking or >15 % increase in DBP. If various forms of hypertension are incorrectly diagnosed the health of the mother and child can be adversely affected.

1. Chronic hypertension: present at booking appointment or prior to 20 weeks gestation.
2. Gestational hypertension: new hypertension present after 20 weeks without significant proteinuria, increased risk of pre-eclampsia in subsequent pregnancies. (Such patients should be advised to take 75 mg aspirin from 12 weeks in future pregnancies).
3. Pre-eclampsia: new hypertension present after 20 weeks with significant proteinuria (>300 mg protein in 24 h urinary collection or >30 mg/mmol in urinary protein:creatinine ratio).

Clinical Assessment

History

Patients are often asymptomatic, but careful evaluation will enable appropriate investigations and management to be undertaken. History taking should have three main aims when assessing a patient with hypertension:

1. To determine if a patient has secondary hypertension which may respond to specific therapies and factors that may be aggravating blood pressure levels and hypertension
2. To detect the presence of target organ damage which may require additional or more aggressive management
3. To identify and correct other risk factors for cardiovascular disease in that patient

Features to increase suspicion of secondary hypertension can be seen in Table 5.3.

Factors that may aggravate blood pressure levels and hypertension

(i) Lifestyle: smoking, diet – high sodium/low dietary fruit and vegetable intake, high alcohol consumption, low levels of physical activity, caffeine intake

TABLE 5.3 Red flags for secondary hypertension	Age of onset <30 years or >60 years
	Family history of hypertension at a young age
	Resistant hypertension (uncontrolled on 3 medications)
	Hypertensive crisis
	Hypokalaemia
	Renal impairment or abnormal U&Es
	Signs and symptoms of secondary cause

(ii) Medications: oral contraceptives, cyclosporine, NSAIDs, glucocorticoids, illicit substances (particularly cocaine and amphetamines) abrupt cessation of antihypertensive medications such as β-blockers

Examination

This provides verifying blood pressure readings, evidence of target organ damage and the opportunity to detect signs of secondary hypertension.

- Record BP, in both arms if appropriate
- Height, weight and body mass index (BMI)
- *Cardiovascular*: radio-femoral delay, elevated JVP, S_3 or S_4, cardiac murmurs, carotid bruits, renal bruits, peripheral pulses (if PVD), peripheral oedema and fluid status
- *Neurological*: fundoscopy for hypertensive retinopathy (see Table 5.4), neurological deficits
- *Abdominal*: unequal kidney size, waist circumference, urinary bladder distension and cushingoid features

TABLE 5.4 Features of hypertensive retinopathy

Grade	Features
I	Tortuous arteries with silver or copper wiring
II	AV nipping
III	Flame haemorrhages, cotton wool spots
IV	Papilloedema

Investigations

A routine panel of investigations should be ordered for all patients with a new diagnosis of hypertension. This will both assess the patients baseline prior to initiation of treatment and to assess target organ damage. In pateints in whom a secondary cause is suspected, further investigations should be requested.

Basic:

- Urine: dipstick for protein, blood and glucose, send urinary albumin:creatinine ratio
- Blood: U&Es, serum total and HDL cholesterol, glucose
- ECG
- Echocardiogram if ECG suggestive of left ventricular hypertrophy

Investigation for Secondary Causes

Renal or reno-vascular disease may be suspected in patients with abnormal urine dip, abdominal bruits, impaired renal function or worsening of renal function with ACE-I or ARBs. Renal causes can be investigated with duplex ultrasound of the kidneys or magnetic resonance angiography.

If the patient is hypokalaemic, causes of hyperaldosteronism (such as Conn's syndrome or adrenal hyperplasia) should be considered. The aldosterone:renin ratio will detect primary aldosteronism, and referral for further investigation can be made.

Patients with features of Cushing's not on exogenous steroids should undergo a dexamethasone suppression test with consideration of further investigations such as plasma ACTH, high dose dexamethasone suppression test and MRI of the pituitary.

Phaeochromocytoma should be suspected in patients with palpitations, flushing, sweating, headaches and decreased gastrointestinal motility. They need immediate investigation with 24 h unrinary collection for metadrenaline and normetadrenaline. Specialist referral is advised as ultimate management involves removal of the tumour.

Hyper and hypothyroidism may both cause hypertension and can easily be excluded with the addition of thyroid function tests in the blood panel if suspected. Acromegaly should be suspected in a patient who is noted to have enlarged facial features, hands and feet, excessive sweating and impaired glucose tolerance and is diagnosed with elevated growth hormone.

Coarctation of the aorta should be suspected with radio-femoral delay and weak femoral pulses. CXR may be suggestive and Doppler or CT aorta will provide a diagnosis.

Obstructive sleep apnoea should be considered in the obese patient with daytime somnolence, loud snoring and increased neck circumference. Polysomnography is the main diagnostic tool.

Significant family history of hypertension in young patients with hypertension in young family members should prompt consideration of referral for genetic analysis to assess for the presence of any monogenetic disorders.

Management

An overview of the update care pathway from NICE and British Hypertension Society can be seen in the 'Hypertension: Quick Reference Guide'.

Targets

Patients should have medications titrated to achieve a clinic blood pressure of <140/90 mmHg, HBMP or ABPM

<135/85 mmHg. Newer studies have recently provided information as to the benefits of treating hypertension in patients aged over 80 years, which includes significant reduction in cardiovascular events, stroke and heart failure. Patients diagnosed with hypertension when aged 80 years or above should have a target clinic BP of <150/90 mmHg, HBPM or ABMP <145/85 mmHg. These higher targets reflect the uncertainty of harms which may be associated with lower blood pressures such as falls.

It is not certain that high risk patient such as those with renal disease and proteinurea, diabetes, history of CVA and IHD benefit from lower BP targets (previously 130/80 mmHg).

Cardiovascular Risk Factor Assessment

Hypertension should trigger full assessment of cardiovascular risk factors using a validated cardiovascular disease risk assessment tool such as the Framingham risk equation. A reduction in all risk factors maximises benefits for patients' future health. It is worth noting that risk assessment tools may underestimate cardiovascular risk in certain groups of patients, and adjustments should be made according to national recommendations.

Lifestyle Advice

Lifestyle interventions should be offered to all patients, particularly to those with borderline hypertension to perhaps delay the need for medications for a few years. Lifestyle alterations have been shown to reduce systolic and diastolic BP and encourages patient ownership of their health with appropriate advice and support from medical professionals including written information and patient support groups. Evidence for lifestyle intervention is not as rigorous as pharmacological interventions and determining if the effects are maintained over longer periods have been difficult to ascertain. Current guidelines produced by collaboration between the British Hypertension Society and NICE recommend the following:

- Maximum of 6 g per day of sodium chloride (2.4 g sodium)
- Moderate alcohol intake (maximum 21 units alcohol per week for males, maximum 14 units per week for women)
- Reduce caffeine consumption
- Advise smoking cessation. Although there is no direct link between smoking and hypertension, it reduces overall cardiovascular risk and reduces mortality and morbidity generally
- Encourage aerobic exercise e.g. 30 min of brisk walking per day. Relaxation therapies with biofeedback have also been proven to lower blood pressure and can be incorporated into lifestyle changes although this is not to be provided by the primary care team
- Dietary advice to increase fruit and vegetable intake and reduced saturated and total fat intake

Pharmacological Therapy

The decision to initiate medication should be carefully considered and the patient counselled adequately to highlight the importance of the need to take medications for life. Each drug will lower BP by approximately 7–8 mmHg although there is wide inter-patient variability in response and in order to meet blood pressure targets some patients will require two or more pharmacological agents (National Institute for Health and Care Excellence 2011a). A summary of most current NICE guidelines can be seen in Fig. 5.1.

Step 1 medication should be initiated in any patient with stage 2 hypertension, and any patient with stage 1 hypertension with target organ damage or established cardiovascular disease or renal disease or diabetes or 10 year cardiovascular risk greater than 20 %. Patients aged over 55 or of African or Caribbean origin of any age should be initially offered a calcium channel blocker. New recommendations state that if

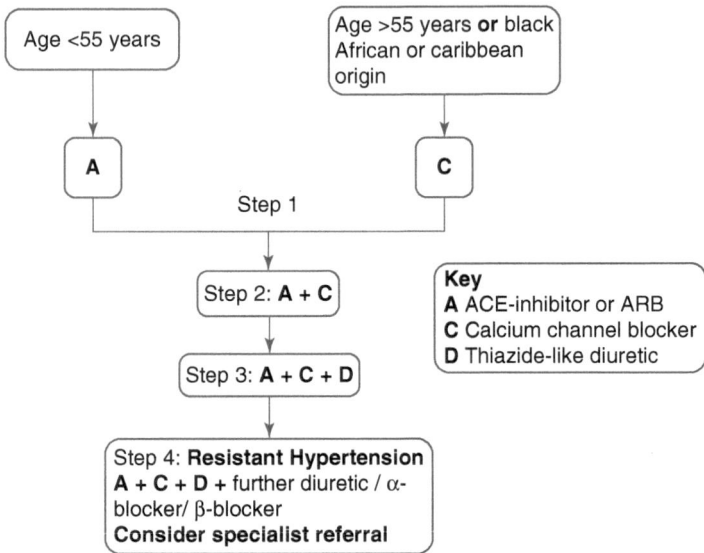

FIGURE 5.1 Summary of pharmacological management of hypertensive patients (Adapted from National Institute for Health and Care Excellence (2011a))

this is not tolerated or evidence of heart failure is present, a thiazide-like diuretic such as indapamide or chlortalidone should be commenced in preference to a conventional thiazide diuretic such as bendroflumethiazide. If patients are currently established on a traditional thiazide diuretic, this should be continued. Beta blockers are not preferred within the current guidelines, but still may have a therapeutic role in young patients intolerant of ACE-inhibitors and ARBs, young women of childbearing age and those with increased sympathetic drive.

In step 2 medication, an ACE inhibitor or ARB with CCB should be offered. In patients with CCB intolerance or evidence of heart failure, a thiazide-like diuretic should be offered instead. Patients of African or Caribbean family origin should be offered an ARB in preference to an ACE inhibitor. If targets are still unmet, ensure compliance with current medication and up-titrate doses to optimum or maximum tolerated before offering step 3 therapies.

If patients do not meet clinic targets of <140/90 mmHg on a combination of three drugs – with one being a diuretic, this is classified as resistant hypertension and requires referral to specialist services (Table 5.5).

Hypertensive Crises

Hypertension is often asymptomatic and chronic in nature. However, patients can present with a hypertensive crisis which is classified as a medical emergency and warrants immediate referral and admission to an inpatient setting for blood pressure lowering medication.

Accelerated hypertension is BP ≥210/130 with target organ damage such as headaches and hypertensive encephalopathy, proteinurea and renal failure, shortness of breath and cardiac failure, visual disturbance and hypertensive retinopathy up to grade 3 (see Table 5.3). Malignant hypertension is as accelerated hypertension with the addition of papilloedema on fundoscopy (grade 4 hypertensive retinopathy).

Blood pressure reduction should aim to reduce blood pressure in a controlled manner to a target of 160/100 mmHg after 6 h of therapy. This minimises risks of morbidity from myocardial infarction and cerebrovascular accidents.

In the presence of acute life threatening organ damage, intravenous medications can be used, however this needs to be done in a level 2 care setting (HDU). Such treatments include sodium nitroprusside, glyceryl trinitrate (particularly with cardiac failure), labetalol (with aortic dissection) and phentolamine (with phaeochromocytoma) and may be preferred according to the respective clinical scenario.

In less urgent circumstances, nifedipine MR 10–20 mg is often used as a first line drug. This can be repeated after 2 h and titrated to a maximum dosage of 20 mg tds. ACE inhibitors and diuretics should be avoided in these circumstances

TABLE 5.5 Common medications in treatment of hypertension

Medication (Class, generic names)	Mechanism of action	Indications	Cautions	Contraindications
ACE-inhibitors captopril, enalapril, lisinopril, ramipril	Decreased angiotensin-II production	Heart failure, LVH, established IHD, T1DM nephropathy	Renal impairment (should be initiated under specialist supervision in those with CKD)	Pregnancy, renovascular disease
ARBs candesartan, irbesartan, losartan, valsartan	Selective inhibition of AT-I receptor	Intolerance of ACE-I, T2DM nephropathy	Renal impairment (should be initiated under specialist supervision in those with CKD)	Pregnancy, renovascular disease
CCBs: Dihydropyridines amlodipine, felodipine, nifedipine MR	Vasodilation and natriuresis	LVH, pregnancy, angina	Tachyarrhythmia, heart failure	
CCBs: Rate limiting diltiazem, verapamil	Negatively inotropic, vasodilation and natriuresis	Angina, SVT	Co-therapy with β-blockers (precipitate heart block)	Heart block, heart failure

Drug class	Mechanism	Indications	Cautions	Contraindications
Thiazide diuretics bendroflumethiazide, hydochlorthiazide	Vasodilation and moderate diuresis	Heart failure	Co-therapy with β-blockers (increased risk of diabetes), can cause hypokalaemia	Gout
Thiazide-like diuretics indapamide, chlortalidone	Vasodilation and moderate diuresis	Heart failure	Co-therapy with β-blockers (increased risk of diabetes), can cause hypokalaemia	Gout
α-blockers doxazosin, prazosin	Alpha-1 receptor antagonists	BPH, resistant hypertension	Postural hypotension	Urinary incontinence
β-blockers atenolol, bisoprolol, metoprolol, sotalol	Suppress plasma renin production, negatively chrono and inotropic	MI, angina, stable heart failure, young women of childbearing age	Co-therapy with thiazide and thiazide-diuretics	Asthma, COPD, heart block, unstable heart failure

as they may precipitate a rapid fall in BP without adequate fluid supplementation.

Further Reading

Craig R, Mindell J, editors. Health survey for England 2012. London: The Health and Social Care Information Centre; 2013.

Hayward C, et al. Drugs in cardiology. Oxford: Oxford University Press; 2011.

Longmore M, et al. Oxford handbook of clinical medicine. Oxford: Oxford University Press; 2008.

National Institute for Health and Care Excellence. Lipid modification CG 67. London: National institute for Health and Care Excellence; 2010.

National Institute for Health and Care Excellence. The clinical management of primary hypertension in adults CG 127. London: National institute for Health and Care Excellence; 2011a.

National Institute for Health and Care Excellence. Hypertension: quick reference guide CG 127. London: National institute for Health and Care Excellence; 2011b.

Royal College of Obstetricians and Gynaecologists. Hypertension in pregnancy: the management of hypertensive disorders during pregnancy. London: Royal College of Obstetricians and Gynaecologists; 2011.

Index

J.C. Kaski et al. (eds.), *Investigating and Managing Common*   143
Cardiovascular Conditions, DOI 10.1007/978-1-4471-6696-2,
© Springer-Verlag London 2015